THE AUTHORS

Rosemary Conley lives in Leicestershire with her husband and business partner, Mike Rimmington, with whom she runs Rosemary Conley Enterprises.

A qualified exercise teacher, Rosemary has worked in the field of slimming and exercise for twenty years, but it was in 1986 that she discovered by accident that low-fat eating led to a leaner body. Forced on to a very low-fat diet as a result of a gallstone problem, not only did Rosemary avoid major surgery but her previously disproportionately large hips and thighs reduced dramatically in size. After extensive research and trials her *Hip and Thigh Diet* was published in 1988 by Arrow Books. This book and its sequel, *Rosemary Conley's Complete Hip and Thigh Diet*, have dominated the bestseller list for four years and have sold in excess of 2 million copies. *Rosemary Conley's Hip and Thigh Diet* has been translated into five languages, including Hebrew and Greek. Subsequent titles, *Hip and Thigh Diet Cookbook*, *Inch Loss Plan*, *Metabolism Booster Diet* and *Whole Body Programme*, have all been instant number 1 bestsellers.

Rosemary has travelled the world promoting her books and her *Hip and Thigh Diet* has been number 1 in New Zealand, Australia, Canada and South Africa. She has appeared on numerous radio and television programmes world-wide, including the Ray Martin Show in Australia and the Wogan Show in the UK. Since 1990 Rosemary has had her own series on network BBC 1 television.

In 1991 her *Whole Body Programme* video was launched by BBC Video. It too became a number 1 bestseller, topping the UK video charts for many months. It is to date the bestselling fitness video ever to have been released in this country. Further of her videos include *Whole Body Programme 2*, *7-Day Workout* and the *Top To Toe Collection*.

Rosemary is now accepted as the leading authority in the UK on weight and inch loss. When asked why she has achieved so much success she says, 'It's simply because my diets and exercises work for ordinary, real people.'

Rosemary is a committed Christian and has a daughter, Dawn, by her first marriage.

Patricia Bourne trained in catering and home economics and ran her own catering business for several years, cooking for occasions ranging from small dinner parties to wedding receptions for over 200 people. She joined the staff of the Tante Marie School of Cookery in 1969 and became Head Teacher eight years later and then Principal in 1981. She is a Fellow of the Cookery and Food Association, a Master Craftsman of the Craft Guild of Chefs and a member of the Surrey Wine and Food Society. Patricia wrote *The Cooks Handbook*, *Tante Marie Book of Traditional French Cookery* and *Sweet Temptation* with Wendy Majerowicz, and since she has retired from teaching has written several other books including *French Bistro Cookery*, *Choice Desserts* and *French Vegetable Cookery*.

D0334031

Rosemary Conley's
New
Hip and Thigh Diet
Cookbook

ROSEMARY CONLEY &
PATRICIA BOURNE

TED SMART

A TED SMART Publication 1997

Arrow Books Limited
20 Vauxhall Bridge Road, London SW1V 2SA

An imprint of Random House UK Ltd

London Melbourne Sydney Auckland Johannesburg
and agencies throughout the world

First published in 1993 by Arrow Books Limited

7 9 10 8

Designed by Roger Walker

ISBN 0 09 921991 3

Printed and bound in Great Britain by
Cox & Wyman Ltd, Reading, Berkshire

Contents

Acknowledgements

I was delighted to be asked to write another cookbook for Rosemary's Hip and Thigh Diet. I have thoroughly enjoyed collaborating with her again and must thank her for all her support.

I also wish to thank our editor Jan Bowmer at Random House for all her help and especially Valerie Buckingham, my copy editor, for all her hard work in editing these pages and her, as always, helpful advice. Without the back-up of people like Jan and Valerie, my task would have been much greater and I have so enjoyed working with them again.

I must also thank friends for allowing me to use their recipes, in particular, Mary Bond, Cicely and Peter Jessop and Marian Kenward.

My children Alison Russell, Neil Bourne and Clare Rule have also entered into the spirit of this diet and have created dishes for me to use and to them I give my love and thanks.

I wish to acknowledge my debt to Dave Marriott for the historical information he unearthed for me, and to Giovanni Fontebasso for his help in making the photographs of the boned chicken on which the diagrams are based. Also, my thanks to my son-in-law, Harry Rule and to Barbara Strange for helping me master my new wordprocessor and thus enable me to get this book prepared.

Finally, I must again thank my husband Tony for his patient and continual help and support, not only when writing this book but at all times.

Without my family, colleagues and friends, I would be a much poorer person and I thank you all very much indeed.

Pat Bourne, July 1992

Introduction
by Rosemary Conley

I have to admit that when my first Hip and Thigh Diet book was published in 1988 I did not anticipate the phenomenal effect it would have on the eating habits and the lives of so many people, not only in the UK but across the world. Perhaps even more significant is the fact that my findings indicate that, unlike with other diet programmes, the vast majority of those who seriously follow my diet do in fact maintain their weight loss in the long term. The Hip and Thigh Diet is not a fad diet – it is undoubtedly here to stay.

The reason for this phenomenal success is simple. Not only have dieters actually acquired the body shape they never even dreamed could be theirs but, just as importantly, their old eating habits were re-educated. People are prepared to make long-term changes to their diet to achieve the desired results. It is a classic case of cause and effect. Remove that which does the damage (fat), introduce that which does the good (healthy eating and exercise), and the effect is a low-fat, healthy body. Using this principle, families changed their eating habits of a lifetime and learned to cook without automatically adding fat.

In 1989 my first *Hip and Thigh Diet Cookbook* was published. Another instant number one bestseller, it has proved extraordinarily popular among Hip and Thigh disciples. My co-author of the original cookbook and now this new one is Patricia Bourne. We first met in 1988 after Pat wrote to me explaining that she had been successfully following my diet. As a qualified chef and experienced cookery writer, she suggested that we produce a cookbook together. I was immediately attracted to Pat because she is so much more than just a cookery writer. Not only does she create the most delicious recipes, bringing together exciting combinations of foods that I would never have dreamed of, but she also slips in lots of invaluable advice, tips and general information to ensure that even the novice cook achieves perfect results.

On the instructional side you can learn how to bone a chicken, how to make vegetable pureés, why you shouldn't use the skin of plaice when making fish stock (it makes it bitter) and why you should use only small white mushrooms in white sauces (larger ones will make it grey), plus lots more. Pat has given thought to convenience and economy too by suggesting different types of fish or meat if all varieties are not available to you. There's advice on how to microwave many of the recipes, and tips about deep-freezing.

Use this book as a Hip and Thigh Diet friend. It will help you to learn how to cook low-fat style and give you lots of ideas for adapting or creating your own low-fat recipes. It should become a firm favourite on the cookbook shelf! I am sure you will not only enjoy the many exciting recipes but you will greatly extend your knowledge of cooking.

This *New Hip and Thigh Diet Cookbook* is packed full of gastronomic delights from the exotic to the economical. There is a chapter for vegetarians, a wide choice of family favourites and a mouthwatering selection for all those who enjoy entertaining. In addition there is a delightful selection of low-fat canâpés for that special event.

The Hip and Thigh Diet has become a way of life for me and my family. It is now seven years on from when I originally started to follow this very low-fat diet for health reasons and I have since improved, fine-tuned and expanded the diet to what I believe is its optimum versatility. For instance, in the original diet egg yolks were on the 'forbidden list' because of their comparatively high fat content, although egg whites, which contain no fat, were always allowed freely. However, because of their versatility and their high nutrient value, I now allow a maximum of two eggs per week to be included within the realms of the diet. This has enabled a wider variety of dishes to be included here.

Another food that has enjoyed a reprieve is fatty fish such as mackerel, tuna and salmon. Since the fish oils that they contain are so nutritionally valuable, as long as these foods are consumed in moderation, they will enhance the quality of your diet without any detriment to its effectiveness in shedding those unwanted inches.

You will also notice the inclusion of a tiny amount of oil in the vegetarian recipes and, occasionally, quantities of low-fat hard cheese have been included as a source of protein. Readers of my earlier books will know that oil, whether animal- or vegetable-based, and hard cheese are included on the 'forbidden list', and this rule *still applies* to anyone who is *not* vegetarian. But it must also be understood that I do not at any time recommend a 'no-fat' diet. Such a diet would be unhealthy, since fat forms a valuable part of our daily diet. But my 'low-fat' diet still incorporates sufficient fat within the foods that are recommended to supply the nutrients necessary for good health. Some of this essential fat is found in the leanest cuts of meat and poultry and in fish. Therefore, vegetarians who follow a low-fat diet may be eating too little fat and, with this in mind, I asked Pat to include a small amount of vegetable oil in some of her vegetarian recipes. The amount works out at less than a teaspoonful per person when the food is served. In *this* context, therefore, oil *is* allowed within my low-fat diet, but this does not mean you may add it liberally elsewhere!

However, non-vegetarians who are following my diet and wish to select one of Pat's meat-free recipes may do so as a special occasion. Such an occasional break from the rules will do little harm to the overall effect of the diet, and maintenance dieters certainly need have no hesitation in selecting whichever dish they like from the full selection of recipes included.

For those wishing to embark on a serious weight- and inch-loss campaign, I suggest you refer to my *Complete Hip and Thigh Diet* for the full diet instructions, as it is important to understand these thoroughly. However, the recipes included in this cookbook will offer a greater variety of choice for both Hip and Thigh

Dieters and for those on the Maintenance Programme.

I have received a great number of letters from dieters who boast that they serve Hip and Thigh Diet dishes at their dinner parties and no one guesses it is low-fat cuisine. This book is packed full of just such dishes, whether it be Duck with Oriental Sauce (which includes kumquats and lychees – I always wondered how to use these!), Pheasant with Orange, Chicken Cicelia, Red Bean and Burgundy Casserole, Potato Quiche or Guinness Hot-pot, Pineapple and Lemon Cheesecake or Austrian Apple and Orange Ring – your guests will be begging for more! Accordingly, I have included some suggestions for dinner party menus. The following menus are simply a guide to combining some of the many delicious recipes included within this book. As you experiment with different dishes that appeal to you and your family, I am sure you will be able to form your own menus with confidence. Remember to balance the preparation time available with the tastes of your guests and the availability of the ingredients before making your final selection.

In some instances I have made some suggestions for vegetable or salad accompaniments based on Pat's recommendations. Otherwise you may like to select one of the mouthwatering vegetable or salad recipes included on pages 183 to 206 according to the preparation time you have available, or simply serve new potatoes, peas and carrots!

The menus are listed according to the primary ingredient of the main course: fish, meat, poultry or vegetarian. Mix and match the starters and desserts as you wish and don't forget to include others from the earlier *Hip and Thigh Diet Cookbook* in order to expand your repertoire.

Within these dinner party menus I have attempted to combine recipes to give maximum nutrition and also to balance out the overall calorie and fat content. Some dishes, for example in the vegetarian chapter, are slightly higher in fat that would be recommended when rigidly following the diet, but it is far better that you include these than have cream in your coffee or cheese and biscuits following the meal!

While several of the recipes included in this book are particularly suitable for dinner parties, there are lots more ideas for delicious dishes for everyday life.

NB In selecting your menus, please remember to restrict egg yolks to a maximum of two per person per week, and that red meat also should be served only twice a week.

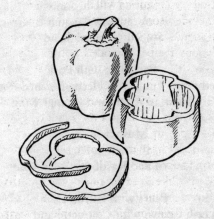

Suggested Dinner Party Menus

FISH MAIN COURSES

Stuffed Mushrooms
Rock Salmon Basquaise
Spiced Tropical Salad
— • —

Pawpaws with Port
Baked Fresh Tuna with Herby Mashed Potatoes
Austrian Apple and Orange Ring
— • —

Mushroom Pâté
Plaice in a Parcel
Lemon and Raspberry Meringue
— • —

Pears with Parma Ham
Florentine Fish Crown with Courgette and Carrot Timbales
Apricot and Ginger Fool
— • —

Grapefruit Surprise
Brochettes of Fish Tandoori
Peach Yogurt Ice
— • —

Côte d'Azur Salad
Fish and Mushroom Timbale
Strawberry and Passion Fruit Pavlova
— • —

Piquant Tomato Jellies
Braised Trout with Crispy Courgettes and Oven Sauté Potatoes
Pineapple and Lemon Cheesecake

Sévigné Tomatoes
Scallops and Monkfish with a Vegetable Tagliatelle
Grapefruit and Kiwi Dessert

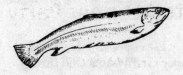

POULTRY AND GAME MAIN COURSES

Tomatoes Beauregard
Chicken Cicelia with broccoli and sweetcorn
Fruit Terrine
— • —
Bacon and Mushroom Roulade
Party Chicken with Gourmet Salad with Kiwi Sauce
Spiced Tropical Salad
— • —
Brussels Sprouts Soup
Chicken with Barbecue Sauce with Oven Sauté Potatoes,
Oriental Cabbage, carrots and sweetcorn
Apple and Mandarin Delight
— • —
Piquant Tomato Jellies
Chicken and Mango Salad
Strawberry and Passion Fruit Pavlova
— • —
Cauliflower, Prawn and Crab Salad
Indonesian Chicken
Peach Yogurt Ice
— • —
Tuna and Tomato Soup
Duck with Oriental Fruit Sauce with Oriental Cabbage,
Farmer's-style Mange-tout and Oven Sauté Potatoes
Pineapple Folly

Stuffed Mushrooms
Venison with Blackcurrants with Dry Roast Potatoes,
Farmer's-style Mange-tout
Lemon and Raspberry Meringue

— • —

Vegetable Broth
Stuffed Turkey Escalopes with Herby Mashed Potatoes,
Celery Paysanne and carrots
Fruit Snowballs

— • —

Bortsch
Sweet 'n' Sour Chicken with rice
Grapefruit and Kiwi Dessert

— • —

Mushroom Pâté
Pheasant with Orange with Dry Roast Potatoes,
Oriental Cabbage, baby sweetcorn and french beans
Peaches Aurora

— • —

Grapefruit Surprise
Guinea Fowl with Lentils, new potatoes,
Farmer's-style Mange-tout and spinach
Grape and Mint Jelly

— • —

Frothy Consommé
Chicken with Prawns with Oven Sauté Potatoes,
courgettes, Brussels sprouts or green beans
Apricot and Ginger Fool

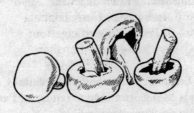

MEAT MAIN COURSES

Frothy Consommé
Apricot Stuffed Lamb with Celeriac Paysanne
Fruit Snowballs
— • —
Cauliflower, Prawn and Crab Salad
Pork and Prunes
Grape and Mint Jelly
— • —
Melon Fans
Beef Carbonnade with Dry Roast Potatoes,
peas, carrots and runner beans
Peaches Aurora

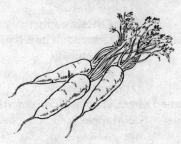

Pawpaws with Port
Ham and Prawn Rolls with mixed salad
Pineapple and Lemon Cheesecake
— • —
Piquant Tomato Jellies
Lamb with Crusty Herb Topping
with Farmer's-style Mange-tout
Orange and Honey Bananas
— • —
Fillets of Mackerel in Cider
Honeyed Pork with Tagliatelle with courgettes and peas
Apple and Mandarin Delight

VEGETARIAN MAIN COURSES

Vegetable Broth
Spinach Roulade with Savoury Brown Rice
Grapefruit and Kiwi Dessert

— • —

Bortsch
Vegetable Couscous
Apricot and Ginger Fool

— • —

Pawpaws with Port
Red Bean and Burgundy Casserole with
Herby Mashed Potatoes and mixed green vegetables
Apple and Mandarin Delight

— • —

Stuffed Mushrooms
Tomato and Vegetable Ring with mixed green salad
Fruit Snowballs

— • —

Hummus
Middle Eastern Pilaff with mixed salad
Pineapple Folly

— • —

$1/2$ melon topped with seedless grapes
Gnocchi Verdi with Fresh Tomato Sauce
Peaches Aurora

— • —

Gourmet Salad with Kiwi Sauce
Spaghetti and Tofu Bolognaise
Peach Yogurt Ice

— • —

Bean and Mushroom Salad
Cottage and Cheddar Cheese Bake with salad and crusty bread
Orange and Honey Bananas

Orange and Onion Salad
Stuffed Aubergines with Chicory and Apple Salad
Lemon and Raspberry Meringues

— • —

Mushrooms à la Greçque
Vegetable and Tofu Salad
Orange and Honey Bananas

— • —

Pawpaws with Port
Mexican Tofu and Bean Stew with
Herby Mashed Potatoes or Potato Quiche
Lemon Sorbet

— • —

Hot Vegetable Salad
Smoked Tofu Kebabs with brown rice
Strawberry and Passion Fruit Pavlova

— • —

Hummus
Italian Vegetable Casserole with Potato Quiche
Apricot and Ginger Fool

— • —

Vegetable Terrine
Provençale Marrow with Potato Quiche or
Herby Mashed Potatoes
Apple and Mandarin Delight

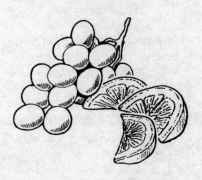

Soups and Starters

The idea of three-course meals on a diet is hard for some people to believe but with Rosemary's amazing *Hip and Thigh Diet* it is possible not only on special occasions but as an everyday occurrence. In this book, I have found some light, interesting and tasty starters and soups to help you vary your diet. Many of them can be used or adapted by vegetarians and vegans and nearly all of them are suitable to serve as light lunch dishes and these have been noted at the start of each recipe.

There are also recipes in other chapters that can be used as starters or lunches. Look particularly at Scallops and Monkfish with a Vegetable Tagliatelle (page 76), Bacon and Mushroom Roulade (page 142), Vegetable Terrine (page 153), and Spinach Roulade (page 159).

The Salad and Vegetable chapter also has plenty of other ideas. The Bean and Mushroom Salad (page 183), Gourmet Salad with Kiwi Sauce (page 184) and the Chicory and Apple Salad (page 186) are all suitable for either occasion and Mushrooms à la Grecque (page 188) are delicious as a starter. Have you ever seen Cocktail Canapés and Savouries in a diet book? I hadn't but I thought 'why not?', and so have included a section which I hope will enable you to enjoy low-fat entertaining.

These are only some of the ideas available to you and I know that you will find others that I hope you will enjoy.

Soups and Starters

> Ⓥ suitable for vegetarians
> Ⓑ budget-conscious recipe
> Ⓠ quick to prepare and cook

STUFFED MUSHROOMS

Serves 4
Cooking time 30–40 minutes
Oven temperature 200°C, 400°F, Gas Mark 6

Vegetarians can also use this recipe by omitting the ham, bacon and prawns, and can, if they wish, substitute them with 50–75g (2–3oz) low-fat grated cheese. This recipe makes an ideal dish for lunch.

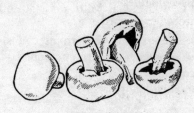

1 medium onion
2 cloves garlic
150 ml (5 floz) cider or stock
4 large flat mushrooms,
approximately 175–225 g (6-8 oz) each
175–225 g (6–8 oz) extra mushrooms
50 g (2 oz) fresh breadcrumbs
100g (4 oz) lean ham or bacon or prawns
150 ml (5 floz) extra stock
salt and black pepper
1/2 teaspoon mixed herbs or Herbes de Provence
2–3 teaspoons Parmesan cheese (maintenance dieters
and vegetarians only)

1. Peel the onion and garlic. Finely chop the onion and crush the garlic. Place in a pan with the cider or stock and simmer gently until tender.
2. Trim and clean all the mushrooms. Remove the stalks from the large mushrooms and chop these finely with the extra mushrooms.

3. When the onions are tender, drain them, reserving the cooking liquor. Mix the chopped mushrooms with the onions, breadcrumbs and garlic. Trim any fat from the ham or bacon and cut into thin strips. Cook the bacon for 2–3 minutes in the reserved cooking liquor. Again, reserve the liquor. Mix the ham, bacon or prawns into the chopped mushroom mixture and season to taste with salt, black pepper and mixed herbs or Herbes de Provence. Pile on top of the large mushrooms, place in a baking dish and pour the reserved cooking liquor and the extra stock into the dish. Cover with aluminium foil or a lid and cook in a preheated oven at 200°C, 400°F, Gas Mark 6 for 30–40 minutes until the large mushrooms are tender.

4. Maintenance dieters and vegetarians can sprinkle a little Parmesan cheese over each mushroom about 10 minutes before the end of the cooking time.

5. Serve hot on individual plates.

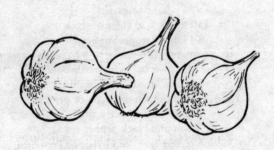

CAULIFLOWER, PRAWN AND CRAB SALAD

Serves 4

This recipe can also be served as a lunch dish.

1 small cauliflower
100–175 g (4–6 oz) white crab meat
4–5 tablespoons Low-fat Salad Cream (page 238)
(or 2 tablespoons low-fat fromage frais or low-fat natural yogurt
mixed with 2 tablespoons reduced-oil salad dressing,
e.g. Waistline or Weight Watchers)
100–175 g (4–6 oz) shelled prawns
chopped fennel, chervil or parsley, to garnish

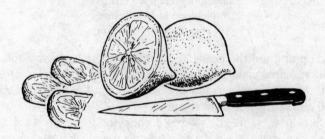

1. Trim the cauliflower and break it into small florets. Cook in boiling, salted water for 7–8 minutes until they are just tender but still have a little bite to them. Drain and chill under cold running water until completely cold (page 246). Drain well again and if necessary lay them on kitchen paper to dry.
2. Mix the cauliflower carefully with the crab meat and sufficient dressing to coat.
3. Pile the mixture into the centre of a round dish or individual dishes and sprinkle the prawns and chopped herbs over.
4. Serve chilled.

CÔTE D'AZUR SALAD

Serves 4

Bought sachets of bouquet garni would be too powerful for this dish so just tie together with string a small piece of celery (the leafy part will do), a few parsley stalks and a bay leaf.

This dish is suitable for lunch. Vegetarians can omit the ham and substitute low-fat cheese.

450 g (1 lb) french beans
450 g (1 lb) ripe tomatoes
2–3 cloves garlic or 1–2 teaspoons garlic paste
1 bouquet garni, see above
salt and black pepper
1 tablespoon capers
1 tablespoon chopped tarragon
1 tablespoon chopped chives
50–75 g (2–3 oz) lean ham

1. Top and tail the beans and cut into short lengths. Cook in boiling, salted water for 4–5 minutes or until just tender. Drain well then chill under cold running water until quite cold. Drain well and refrigerate until required.
2. Skin (page 246), de-seed and chop the tomatoes. Peel and crush the garlic. Place the tomatoes in a pan with the bouquet garni and the garlic. Season lightly with salt and black pepper and cook gently for 7–10 minutes until the tomatoes have reduced to a sauce. Leave until cold and then remove the bouquet garni.
3. Chop the capers and mix into the sauce with most of the chopped tarragon and chives. Trim any fat off the ham and then cut into thin strips before adding to the mixture. Check the seasoning.
4. Pile the beans in a dish and pour the sauce over. Sprinkle the remainder of the herbs over the top.
5. Serve chilled.

SÈVIGNÉ TOMATOES

Serves 4

Since the start of traditional French cookery, chefs have honoured well-known people by naming dishes after them. The best example of this is Peach Melba named by Escoffier at the Savoy Hotel in London after Dame Nellie Melba. Madame de Sèvigné lived in Paris in the 17th century and is famous for the letters she wrote to her daughter over 25 years (1600 of them) which give a vivid account of the history of that time. This dish is a variation on one of those created in her name. I ate it on holiday in France one year and decided to keep the original name. If you prefer to call it Tomatoes Stuffed with Chicken, it will taste just as good. It makes an ideal lunch dish.

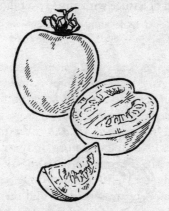

4 large tomatoes (about the size of Golden Delicious apples)
salt and black pepper
100 g (4 oz) mushrooms
150 ml (5 fl oz) chicken stock
½ small green pepper
175–225 g (6–8 oz) diced cold chicken or turkey
4 tablespoons Low-fat Salad Cream (page 238)
a few lettuce leaves, to serve

---

1. If you wish, skin the tomatoes first (page 246). Place the tomatoes stalk side down on a board and cut a slice off the top of each. Reserve these slices. Scoop out the seeds with a ballcutter or teaspoon and season the insides lightly with salt and black pepper. Turn upside down on a wire rack for 20–30 minutes to drain.

2. Wash, trim and thinly slice the mushrooms. Cook them in the stock for 4–5 minutes until just cooked. Remove from the stock and drain well.

3. Remove the stalk, core and seeds from the pepper. Cut into small dice.

4. Mix the mushrooms, chicken and the green pepper together with the Low-fat Salad Cream.

5. Fill each tomato with the mixture, piling it up. Replace the lids at an angle.

6. Serve on a bed of lettuce with any extra filling piled in the centre of the dish.

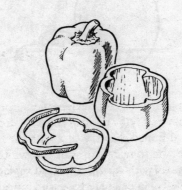

TOMATOES BEAUREGARD

Serves 4

Like the previous recipe, this is a variation of a dish named after a well-known personality. Pierre Beauregard was a general in the Confederate Army during the American Civil War. A similar dish is also named after the state of Monaco in the South of France. This also makes a good dish for lunch.

4 large tomatoes (about the size of Golden Delicious apples)
1 x 225 g (8 oz) can of tuna fish in brine
2 hard-boiled eggs
3–4 tablespoons Low-fat Salad Cream (page 238)
salt and white pepper
a few lettuce leaves, to serve

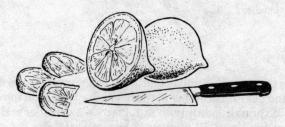

1. Prepare the tomatoes as for Sèvigné Tomatoes (opposite).
2. Drain the tuna and flake the fish coarsely in a bowl.
3. Chop the hard-boiled eggs and mix with the fish and Low-fat Salad Cream. Season to taste with salt and white pepper.
4. Fill the tomatoes with the mixture and replace the lids at an angle. Serve chilled on a bed of lettuce with any extra filling piled in the centre of the dish.

MELON FANS

Serves 4

½ cucumber
salt
1 small honeydew or cantaloupe melon
2 large tomatoes
175–225 g (6–8 oz) peeled prawns
4–5 tablespoons Oil-free Vinaigrette (page 239)
white pepper
chopped fresh basil or chervil

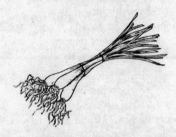

1. Peel the cucumber and cut into half lengthways. Scoop out the seeds and cut the cucumber in short lengths; then cut it into small dice and sprinkle lightly with salt. Place in a colander and allow to drain for about 30 minutes. Rinse well and dry on kitchen paper.
2. Cut the melon in half across the middle and then in half again. Remove the seeds and cut off the skin. Cut the melon in slices almost through to the point. Press down lightly to form a fan. Place on individual small plates with the point towards the centre.
3. Skin (page 246) and de-seed the tomatoes then chop them roughly. Mix the tomatoes with the cucumber and the prawns. Stir in the Oil-free Vinaigrette. Season to taste with salt and pepper and mix in the chopped herbs. Pile the mixture at the point of each melon fan. Cover with food wrap and refrigerate until served.

MUSHROOM PÂTÉ

Serves 6 as a starter or 4–5 as a main dish
Oven 180°C, 350°F, Gas Mark 4

This is another dish very suitable for vegetarians, both as a starter and as a main course. It can also be served for lunch with a salad. Choose either of the Tomato Sauces on pages 235–236 to serve with it.

1 onion
2 cloves garlic
150 ml (5 fl oz) chicken or vegetable stock
450 g (1 lb) button mushrooms
50 g (2 oz) fresh breadcrumbs
a pinch of nutmeg
salt and black pepper
2 egg whites
lemon, to serve
Tomato Sauce (pages 235 and 236), to serve

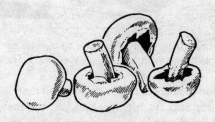

1. Peel and finely chop the onion. Peel and crush the garlic. Place the onion and garlic in a small pan with the stock and cook for 6–7 minutes until almost tender.

2. In the meantime, trim, clean and roughly chop the mushrooms. Add to the pan and cook until the mixture is dry. Transfer the mushrooms to a food processor or liquidiser and purée. If a liquidiser is used, it may be necessary to add an extra egg white at this point.

3. Transfer the purée to a large bowl and mix with the breadcrumbs. Season to taste with nutmeg, salt and pepper. Take care if a stockcube has been used for making the stock as this should season the mushrooms sufficiently.

4. Whisk the egg whites until they stand in stiff peaks and fold into the mushroom mixture in 2–3 batches. Pour into a non-stick 450 g (1 lb) loaf tin or into a loaf tin lined with lightly oiled greaseproof paper. Place the tin in a roasting tin of hot water and cook in a preheated oven at 180°C, 350°F, Gas Mark 4 for 30–40 minutes, until the pâté is firm like a sponge and is coming away from the sides of the tin.

5. Serve hot garnished with thin slices of lemon and Tomato Sauce, or cold with salad.

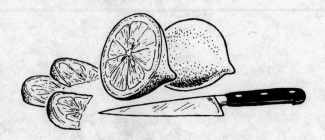

PAWPAWS WITH PORT

Serves 4

2 ripe pawpaws
1 lime
white pepper
225 ml (7½ fl oz) port

1. Cut the pawpaws in half and scoop out the seeds with a small teaspoon.
2. Squeeze the juice from the lime and brush over each pawpaw half. Season lightly with white pepper.
3. Pour the port into the centre of each pawpaw half. Cover with food wrap and refrigerate for about 1 hour.
4. Serve well chilled.

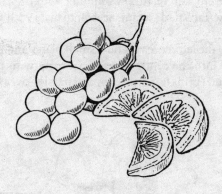

GRAPEFRUIT SURPRISE

Serves 4

Vegetarians can substitute Feta cheese (make sure it is fresh and not bottled in oil) for chicken or turkey. This is a suitable recipe for lunch.

2 large grapefruit
175 g (6 oz) cooked chicken or turkey
3 tablespoons chopped celery
2–3 tablespoons Low-fat Salad Cream (page 238)
salt and white pepper
a few lettuce leaves, to serve
chopped parsley, to garnish

1. Cut the peel and pith from the grapefruit and then cut out the segments from between the membranes.
2. Dice the chicken or turkey and mix with the chopped celery and the Low-fat Salad Cream. Season to taste with salt and white pepper.
3. Arrange the lettuce leaves on 4 small plates and pile the chicken mixture into the centre of each. Garnish with the grapefruit segments and sprinkle a little chopped parsley over the top. Serve chilled.

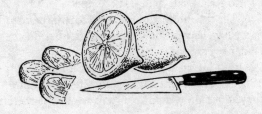

FILLETS OF MACKEREL IN CIDER

Serves 4
Cooking time 20–30 minutes
Oven 180°C, 350°F, Gas Mark 4

Herrings can also be cooked by this method. The dish can be eaten at lunch with a salad.

4 small mackerel
salt and black pepper
1 onion
6 peppercorns
1–2 bay leaves
a few parsley stalks
300 ml (10 fl oz) dry cider

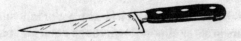

1. Fillet the mackerel or ask your fishmonger to do this for you. Cut off the head, the fins and the tail and cut the fish into individual fillets. Wash well and roll up from the head end. Skewer each one, if you wish, with a cocktail stick. Place in an ovenproof dish and season with salt and black pepper.
2. Peel and slice the onion and place on top of the fish. Tuck the peppercorns, bay leaves and parsley stalks beside the fish and pour the cider over.
3. Cover with a lid or aluminium foil and bake in a preheated oven at 180°C, 350°F, Gas Mark 4 for 20–30 minutes. Leave in the cooking liquor until cold then remove the peppercorns, bay leaves and parsley stalks.
4. Serve cold with salad.

PEARS WITH PARMA HAM

Serves 4

The Italians have a saying which roughly translated says, 'Don't tell the peasants about this dish, it's too good for them to eat.' Do try it as an alternative to the usual melon.

2 large ripe pears
1 lemon or lime
a few lettuce leaves, to serve
4 wafer-thin slices of Parma ham (page 37)
1 small orange, to garnish

1. Peel the pears, cut them in half and remove the cores with a ballcutter or a small teaspoon.
2. Squeeze the juice from the lemon or lime and brush over the pears.
3. Arrange the lettuce leaves on a large plate or individual plates. Cut the pears in slices almost down to the point and place on the lettuce. Press down lightly to fan the slices out.
4. Trim any fat from the Parma ham and place a slice lightly over each pear half so that it wrinkles slightly.
5. Decorate with the orange if you wish by using a canelle knife (page 245) and cut the oranges into thin slices. Cut each slice in half and use to garnish the pears.
6. Chill until required.

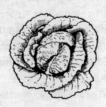

PIQUANT TOMATO JELLIES

Serves 5–6

Vegetarians can make this dish and use a gelatine substitute.

450 g (1 lb) ripe tomatoes
2 small onions
1–2 cloves garlic or ¹/₂–1 teaspoon garlic paste
1 bay leaf
1 teaspoon sugar
celery salt
1 x 11 g (¹/₂ oz) sachet of gelatine
1 tablespoon Worcestershire sauce
2 teaspoons white wine vinegar
2–3 tablespoons lemon juice
salt and white pepper
watercress, to garnish

1. Skin (page 246) the tomatoes and chop coarsely. Peel and finely chop the onion. Peel and crush the garlic. Place them all together in a pan with the bay leaf and sugar and season to taste with the celery salt. Cook gently over a low heat until the onion is tender.
2. Sprinkle the gelatine on to 3 tablespoons water in a small bowl. When it has become soft, place over a pan of hot water until the gelatine has dissolved.
3. In the meantime, when the onions are cooked, remove the bay leaf and purée the tomato mixture then sieve to remove the tomato seeds.
4. Add the gelatine, Worcestershire sauce, white wine vinegar and 2 tablespoons lemon juice to the tomato purée and make up the quantity to 600 ml (1 pint) with water. Check the seasoning and add more celery salt or table salt, white pepper, Worcestershire sauce, lemon juice or sugar to taste.
5. Pour into wetted individual rings or ramekin dishes and leave to set.
6. Turn out on to individual plates and garnish with watercress.

COCKTAIL CANÂPÉS AND SAVOURIES

Cocktail parties can be the death of any diet with crisps, nuts, pastries and cheese abounding. Drinks are easier to control with spritzers and other low-calorie drinks but what can you give your guests that you can also eat? With the following selection you can provide a good variety which your friends can enjoy and you will also be able (with care) to indulge yourself. Take care not to eat too many of the bread- and grissini-based canâpés: although we don't count calories on the Hip and Thigh Diet it is best to avoid too many starchy titbits. Also, have plenty of crudités around, with or without dips. Everyone enjoys crunching on them and they are healthy too.

COCKTAIL CANÂPÉS

100 g (4 oz) quark or other low-fat soft cheese will make 30–36. For the bases use white or brown bread or toast or rye bread cut into 2.5 cm (1 inch) circles or squares. Mix the following flavours with the quark or other low-fat soft cheese. Pipe or spoon onto the prepared bases and top with the chosen garnishes.

1. Spicy Cheese and Grapes. Blend in horseradish relish and seasoning to suit your own taste. Top with half a black grape.

2. Curry and Mango. Blend a little curry powder and the juice of mango chutney into the cheese. Top with a diamond cut from the mango in the chutney.

3. Russian Style. Mix the cheese with a little grated onion and top with black or red lumpfish roe. If you prefer a less expensive version of this canâpé, top each one with a slice of gherkin.

4. Tomato Flavoured. Mix tomato ketchup into the cheese. Top with a cocktail onion.

5. Fruity. Use plain quark or other low-fat soft cheese. Top with a cocktail cherry or mandarin slice (fresh or canned in natural juice). Dry both fruits well on kitchen paper before using. These are particularly good when made with rye bread.

6. Cut 2 cm (³/4 inch) long rectangles of brown bread. Cover with smoked salmon or smoked trout and top with a short length of asparagus.

COCKTAIL SAVOURIES

A mixture of ham, Parma ham and smoked salmon or sliced smoked pink trout can be used. Use thinly cut ham and if you can buy your Parma ham from an Italian shop you will find it is sliced much thinner than the ham you buy in packets or at the delicatessen counter at the supermarket. Cut the ham or smoked salmon into 1 cm (¹/2 inch) strips. You will find 100 g (4 oz) will make 30–40.

To make a Savoury Hedgehog prepare a selection of the following and put on to cocktail sticks. Stick them into a grapefruit half or a potato wrapped in aluminium foil.

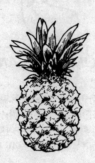

1. Ham wrapped around pineapple (fresh or canned in natural juice).
2. Ham with chunks of gherkin.
3. Ham or smoked salmon with cocktail onions.
4. Parma ham with melon balls or dice.
5. Two rolls of ham, Parma ham or smoked salmon; or mix the ham and Parma ham together.
6. Smoked salmon or trout with prawns.
7. Two or three prawns.

GRISSINI STICKS

Break the grissini sticks into 3–4 pieces. Spread a little quark or other low-fat soft cheese on to the top 2.5 cm (1 inch) and wrap a strip of ham, Parma ham or smoked salmon around each one. Dip a few in poppy seeds for contrast. Stand the completed grissini sticks in small tumblers.

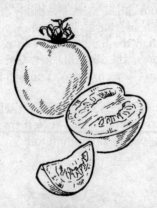

STUFFED TOMATOES AND CELERY

Buy very small tomatoes or cut slightly larger ones in half. Cut a small slice off the top of small tomatoes. Reserve the lids. Scoop the seeds out of the tomatoes and season the insides lightly with salt and pepper. Cut the celery into 4 cm (1¹/2 inch) lengths. Pipe in the following fillings.

1. Purée equal quantities of cottage cheese and tuna (in brine), tinned salmon or smoked mackerel. Season and add a little Tabasco or other chilli sauce if you wish. Replace the lids of tomatoes at a slight angle if you like or top the tomatoes and the celery with a curly piece of smoked salmon, a little lumpfish roe, a slice of gherkin or a little paprika.

2. Blend cottage cheese with grated onion and top with a prawn or two.

3. The toppings for the canâpés (page 36) can also be used.

CRUDITÉS

You may like to serve a dip or two with your crudités.
1. Drain a 350 g (12 oz) can of asparagus spears. Purée with 225 g (8 oz) cottage cheese until smooth. Season to taste.
2. Mix quark or other low-fat soft cheese or low-fat cottage cheese with grated onion and chives.
3. Use the recipe for cottage cheese and tuna opposite.
4. Crush 2–3 cloves of garlic or use 1–1½ teaspoons of garlic paste. Mix with 225 g (8 oz) low-fat natural fromage frais or cottage cheese and stir in 1 tablespoon chopped chives. Season to taste.

CRISPY POTATO SKINS

1 kg (2 lb) medium-sized old potatoes
1 teaspoon oil
salt and black pepper

1. Cut the potatoes into even wedges and cook in boiling, salted water for 7–8 minutes until almost tender.
2. Scoop out the potato flesh. (Mash this while it is hot and use for another recipe such as Smoky Fish and Vegetable Pie (page 59).)
3. In the meantime, heat the oil on a baking tray in a preheated oven at 220°C, 425°F, Gas Mark 7. Toss the potato skins in the oil and cook for 20–25 minutes until they are crisp. Season with salt and pepper (rock salt is particularly good) and serve with the garlic dip above.

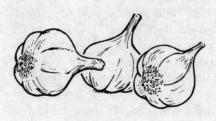

BRUSSELS SPROUTS SOUP

Serves 5–6

This soup is a good way to use large or overblown Brussels sprouts.

450 g (1 lb) Brussels sprouts
1 leek
2 sticks celery
50 g (2 oz) parsnips
100 g (4 oz) carrots
2 medium onions
1 litre (1¾ pints) ham or chicken stock
salt and white pepper
2–3 tablespoons low-fat fromage frais or
low-fat natural yogurt, to garnish

1. Trim the Brussels sprouts and cook in boiling, salted water for 7–8 minutes. Drain, then chill under cold running water until completely cold (page 246).
2. Trim and wash the leek and celery and peel the other vegetables. Dice all the vegetables and place in a pan with the Brussels sprouts. Add the stock and season to taste. Very little salt will be needed if ham stock has been used. Bring to the boil and simmer for 20–25 minutes.
3. Purée the soup in a food processor or liquidiser.
4. Serve hot and garnish the top of each bowl with a swirl of fromage frais or natural yogurt.

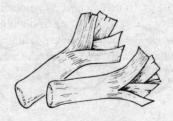

VEGETABLE BROTH

This soup is so easy to make that it is worth while making this quantity and freezing some for another time.

Serves 6–8

225 g (8 oz) onions
225 g (8 oz) carrots
225 g (8 oz) celery
1 x 400 g (14 oz) can chopped tomatoes
1.75 litres (3 pints) chicken or vegetable stock
2 tablespoons tomato purée
50 g (2 oz) pearl barley or 1 x 225 g (8 oz) can baked beans
1–2 teaspoons ground coriander
225 g (8 oz) courgettes
100 g (4 oz) frozen peas or french beans
100 g (4 oz) frozen sweetcorn
salt and pepper

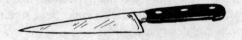

1. Peel the onions and carrots and trim the celery. Cut into small dice. Place in a pan with the tinned tomatoes, stock, tomato purée, pearl barley and add coriander to taste. Season lightly and simmer for 40–50 minutes or until the pearl barley is tender. If pearl barley is not used, simmer for 15–20 minutes.
2. In the meantime, trim and dice the courgettes and add to the pan with the peas or french beans, sweetcorn and the baked beans (if used). Bring to the boil again and simmer for a further 5–6 minutes until all the vegetables are tender. Check the seasoning and add more coriander if required, then pour into a hot soup tureen. Serve hot.

TUNA AND TOMATO SOUP

Serves 4–6

For the best flavour use a really good chicken stock. Poach a chicken (see Indonesian Chicken, page 97) for salads and other made-up dishes and freeze the stock until you need it.

1 litre (1³/4 pints) chicken stock
3 medium onions
3 sticks celery
1 x 400 g (14 oz) can chopped tomatoes
salt and black pepper
1 x 200 g (7 oz) can tuna in brine
100 g (4 oz) button mushrooms
freshly chopped basil or parsley, to garnish

1. Skim any fat from the stock and place it in a large saucepan.
2. Peel the onions and clean the celery and cut both into small dice. Place in the stock with the canned tomatoes and their juice. Season to taste with salt and black pepper and simmer gently until the onions and celery are tender.
3. Drain the tuna and flake into moderately small pieces. Trim, clean and slice the mushrooms.
4. When the vegetables are almost tender, add the mushrooms and cook for another 5–8 minutes then add the tuna. Check the seasoning and pour into a hot soup tureen. Sprinkle a little chopped basil or parsley over just before serving. Serve hot.

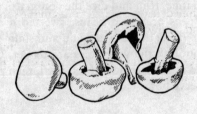

BORTSCH

Serves 4–5

The vinegar used in this recipe is essential to preserve the deep red colour of the beetroot. If it is not used the beetroot loses its colour and looks insipid.

450 g (1 lb) raw beetroot
2 large onions
2 large carrots
2 cloves garlic
3 sticks celery
1.2 litres (2 pints) vegetable or chicken stock
2 tablespoons white wine vinegar or cider vinegar
2 tablespoons tomato purée
salt and black pepper
a little sugar (optional)
4 tablespoons low-fat fromage frais or low-fat natural yogurt

1. Peel the beetroot, onion, carrots and garlic and trim the celery. Grate the beetroot, onion, carrots and celery coarsely and crush the garlic. Place in a pan with the stock, vinegar and tomato purée. Season lightly with salt and black pepper. Bring to the boil and simmer for about 20 minutes until the vegetables are tender.
2. Taste and adjust the seasoning, adding a little sugar if desired.
3. To serve hot, the soup can either be strained or the vegetables can be left in the soup.
4. To serve chilled, leave the vegetables in the soup until it is cold then strain and chill well.
5. Serve either hot or cold in individual soup bowls and pour a spoonful of fromage frais or yogurt on top of each one just before taking to the table.

FROTHY CONSOMMÉ

Serves 4

2 teaspoons gelatine
1 x 400 g (14 oz) can consommé
2 tablespoons sherry
225 g (8 oz) quark or other low-fat soft cheese
salt and white pepper
a few chopped chives, to garnish

1. Pour 2 tablespoons cold water into a small bowl and sprinkle the gelatine on top. Leave to soften then place the bowl over a pan of hot water until the gelatine has dissolved.
2. Stir the gelatine into the consommé and add the sherry. Chill until it is on the point of setting lightly (page 245).
3. Place the consommé and quark or low-fat soft cheese into a food processor or liquidiser and purée until smooth or blend the cheese into the consommé with a hand-held electric whisk or a balloon whisk.
4. Season to taste with salt and white pepper and pour into individual glasses and chill until lightly set. Sprinkle a few chopped chives over the top of each one just before serving.

Fish

In this book, as in the last one, I have tried to use as many different types of fish as possible and you will find that most of the recipes can be adapted to use whichever fish you prefer. I have included rock salmon, a fish seldom used in recipes but it is economical and tasty. Fresh tuna is used widely on the continent and is now often seen in the fishmongers in this country. Do try it if you get the opportunity. It has a dark red flesh which pales while it is cooking. It is really most delicious and, rather like salmon, the fresh fish is totally different from the tinned. Now that Rosemary allows a little oily fish in the diet, I have also included mackerel. Do try the St Clement's Mackerel (page 66). In France, a gooseberry sauce is often served with mackerel and, in my recipe, the unusual combination of mackerel and orange marmalade really do complement each other as the sweet sharpness of the marmalade goes so well with the rich flesh of the mackerel.

There are recipes here for every occasion from simple family meals to special dinners. Do try them all, fish is so good on any diet but particularly on the Hip and Thigh Diet.

Fish

Ⓥ suitable for vegetarians
Ⓑ budget-conscious recipe
Ⓠ quick to prepare and cook

PLAICE IN A PARCEL

Serves 4
Cooking time 15–20 minutes

Cod or haddock steaks or fillets can also be used for this recipe but will take 25–30 minutes to cook. If you wish to alter this recipe to serve one or two, divide the main ingredients into the required amount but do use the full amount of wine or cider used to cook the vegetables, then boil the sauce until it is a coating consistency before pouring it over the fish.

8 x 100–150 g (3–4 oz) single fillets of plaice
2 sticks celery
1 small green pepper
100 g (4 oz) mushrooms
1 onion
150 ml (5 fl oz) white wine or cider
1 tablespoon tomato purée
salt and white pepper

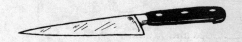

1. Remove the skin from each fillet of plaice or ask your fish-monger to do this for you. Scrape or cut away any black membranes. Cover and refrigerate until required.
2. Trim and finely chop the celery. Remove the stalk, seeds and pith from the pepper and cut into small dice. Trim, clean and finely slice the mushrooms. Peel and finely chop the onion.
3. Place the onion and celery in a small pan with the white wine or cider. Cook gently for 4–5 minutes then add the chopped pepper. Continue cooking for a further minute or two then add the mushrooms and tomato purée. Season to taste.

4. Spread a little sauce on the skin side of each fillet of plaice and roll up. Place two fillets in a square of aluminium foil. Prepare the other fillets in the same way and pour the remainder of the sauce evenly over each one. Fold up and seal the packets and place in a steamer over a pan of boiling water for 15–20 minutes.

5. To serve, place a foil parcel on each plate or individual serving dish and open at the table so that the full flavour is retained.

MICROWAVE
Can be microwaved wrapped in greaseproof paper not aluminium foil or can be cooked in a covered dish.

SUGGESTED VEGETABLES
New or mashed potatoes and any green vegetable.

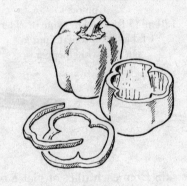

ROCK SALMON BASQUAISE

Serves 4
Cooking time 30–35 minutes
Oven 180°C, 350°F, Gas Mark 4

Other firm white fish such as monkfish, halibut or cod can be used in place of rock salmon if you wish.

450–550 g (1–1¼ lb) rock salmon
350 g (12 oz) onions
2 cloves garlic
150 ml (5 fl oz) fish stock (page 69)
150 ml (5 fl oz) white wine or cider or extra fish stock
1 tablespoon tomato purée
salt and white pepper
¼ teaspoon sweet paprika
1 teaspoon arrowroot
chopped parsley, to garnish
1 lemon, to garnish

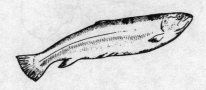

1. Cut the rock salmon into evenly sized pieces. Cover and refrigerate until required.
2. Peel and finely chop the onions. Peel and crush the garlic. Place the onions and garlic in a heatproof dish with the fish stock and white wine or cider. Place over a gentle heat and simmer until the onions are almost tender. Stir in the tomato purée and season with salt, pepper and the sweet paprika. Add the fish to the dish, bring to the boil, cover and place in a preheated oven 180°C 350°F, Gas Mark 4 for 30–35 minutes or until the fish and onions are cooked.

3. Check the seasoning and pile the fish into a hot serving dish. Mix the arrowroot with a little water and add to the liquor in the cooking dish. Bring to the boil, stirring all the time. Check the seasoning and the consistency, adding a little stock, wine or cider if necessary to give a coating consistency. Pour the sauce over the fish. Sprinkle chopped parsley over just before serving and garnish the dish with lemon wedges.

MICROWAVE
Can be microwaved.

SUGGESTED VEGETABLES
Rice, or new or mashed potatoes.
Carrots, broccoli, peas or beans.

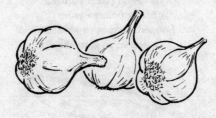

SMOKED HADDOCK CHOWDER

Serves 4
Cooking time 20–25 minutes

450 g (1 lb) small new or small firm old potatoes
450 g (1 lb) smoked haddock
100 g (4 oz) lean back bacon
300 ml (10 fl oz) skimmed milk
150 ml (5 fl oz) fish or chicken stock
75 g (3 oz) red and green peppers, without pith and seeds
175 g (6 oz) canned or frozen sweetcorn
75 g (3 oz) frozen peas
2 tablespoons tomato ketchup
white pepper
2 teaspoons arrowroot
2 tablespoons low-fat fromage frais, quark or
other low-fat soft cheese
100 g (4 oz) peeled prawns, optional
chopped parsley, to garnish

1. Peel the potatoes and cook in boiling, salted water for 10 minutes, then drain and slice thickly.
2. Remove the skin and any bones from the smoked haddock. Remove any fat from the bacon and cut into strips or dice. Place the fish and the bacon in a pan with the milk and stock. You will find an aluminium or non-stick pan better than stainless steel as the milk tends to stick less in these types of pan. Cook for 5–6 minutes until the fish is only just cooked. Remove the fish and bacon from the pan and break the fish into large pieces. Reserve.
3. Cut the peppers into small dice. When the potatoes are ready, add them to the milk with the peppers, sweetcorn and peas. Cover and simmer gently until the potatoes and peppers are tender. Stir occasionally to prevent them sticking to the bottom of the pan.
4. Stir in the tomato ketchup and season with white pepper. There should be no need to add salt as the liquid will be salty

enough from the fish. Bring to the boil. Mix the arrowroot with a little water and add to the pan. Bring to the boil once again, stirring all the time. Take care to stir gently so that the potatoes do not break up.

5. Pour a little of the sauce without any potatoes into a small bowl and whisk in the fromage frais, quark or other low-fat soft cheese. Return this to the pan and add the smoked haddock, and the prawns (if used). Heat through gently and pour into a hot serving dish. Sprinkle chopped parsley over just before serving.

MICROWAVE
Could be microwaved but quicker to cook conventionally. Do not microwave when heating the fromage frais or quark. Follow the conventional recipe for step 5.

SUGGESTED VEGETABLES
This is a complete meal; no extra vegetables are required but a salad could be served after if you wish.

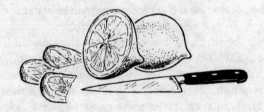

BAKED FRESH TUNA

Fresh tuna is available from many supermarkets and fishmongers. It has a firm meaty flesh and is delicious to eat. If you cannot obtain fresh tuna this recipe can be made with any firm white fish such as cod or haddock. Tuna can also be grilled.

Serves 4
Cooking time 50–60 minutes
Oven 220°C, 425°F, Gas Mark 7

2 medium red peppers
225 g (8 oz) onions
3 cloves garlic or 1½ teaspoons garlic paste
450 g (1 lb) fresh tomatoes or 1 x 400g (14 oz) can chopped tomatoes
150 ml (5 fl oz) fish stock (page 69)
(only required if fresh tomatoes are used)
salt and black pepper
1 tablespoon sweet paprika
2 tablespoons chopped parsley
4 x 175–200 g (6–7 oz) fresh tuna steaks
175 g (6 oz) button mushrooms
extra chopped parsley, to garnish

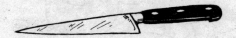

1. Remove the stalk, pith and seeds from the peppers. Peel the onions and garlic. Peel (page 246) and de-seed the fresh tomatoes. Chop the peppers, onions and fresh tomatoes and crush the garlic. Place them in a pan with the fish stock. If canned tomatoes are used, omit the fish stock and add the canned tomatoes and their juice to the pan. Season to taste with salt and black pepper. Bring to the boil and simmer until the onions are almost tender. Check the seasoning and add the paprika and chopped parsley.

2. Place the tuna steaks in a ovenproof dish and pour the sauce over. Cover with a lid or aluminium foil and cook in a preheated oven 220°C, 425°F, Gas Mark 7 for 30 minutes.

3. Clean, trim and slice the mushrooms. Stir into the tomato sauce and continue cooking (uncovered) for a further 10–15 minutes.

4. Sprinkle a little chopped parsley over the top just before serving.

MICROWAVE
This dish can be microwaved.

SUGGESTED VEGETABLES
Rice, Savoury Brown Rice (page 158), new potatoes,
Herby Mashed Potatoes (page 200), peas, beans,
broccoli, cauliflower, mange-tout or a green salad.

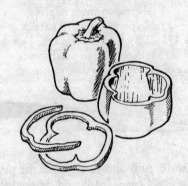

BAKED FISH WITH CURRIED RICE

Serves 4
Cooking time 30–40 minutes
Oven 200°C, 400°F, Gas Mark 6

450–550 g (1–1¼ lb) cod or haddock fillets
2–3 tablespoons lemon juice
salt and white pepper
4 medium onions
300 ml (10 fl oz) Fish Stock (page 69)
100 g (4 oz) lean ham
100 g (4 oz) mushrooms
300 ml (10 fl oz) natural low-fat yogurt
2 tablespoons chopped chives
2 tablespoons chopped parsley
2 teaspoons sweet paprika
5–6 medium tomatoes
3–4 tablespoons fresh breadcrumbs
a little low-fat spread (maintenance dieters only)
175–225 g (6–8 oz) easy-cook rice
50 g (2 oz) raisins
50 g (2 oz) frozen peas
1–2 teaspoons curry powder or to taste

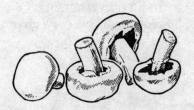

1. Remove the skin from the fish or ask your fishmonger to do this for you. Place the fish in a shallow dish and pour the lemon juice over. Season with salt and white pepper and leave for 15 minutes in the refrigerator.
2. Peel and chop the onions and cook in the fish stock until almost tender. Drain and reserve the fish stock.

3. Remove any fat from the ham and chop coarsely. Trim, clean and thinly slice the mushrooms. Mix half the onions with the ham, mushrooms, yogurt and three-quarters of the chopped chives and parsley. Season to taste and stir in the paprika. Skin (page 246) and slice the tomatoes.

4. Lay the fillets of fish in an oven-to-table dish and cover with the sauce. Arrange the tomatoes on the top and sprinkle the breadcrumbs over. Maintenance dieters only can dot a little low-fat spread on the breadcrumbs. Cook in a preheated oven 200°C, 400°F, Gas Mark 6 for 30–40 minutes.

5. In the meantime cook the rice in boiling, lightly salted water until tender. Pour a little boiling water on the raisins and leave them to soak. Boil the reserved fish stock rapidly to reduce it to about 2 tablespoons and stir in the curry powder. Cook the frozen peas.

6. When the rice is cooked, drain it well and stir into the reduced fish stock with the reserved onions, the raisins and peas. Taste and add more curry powder if necessary. Pile the rice into a hot dish and sprinkle the reserved herbs over just before serving.

MICROWAVE
Do not microwave as the yogurt will toughen.

SUGGESTED VEGETABLES
Beans, broccoli, cauliflower or a green salad.

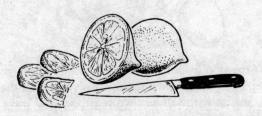

FISHBURGERS

Serves 4
Cooking time 15–20 minutes
Oven 200°C, 400°F, Gas Mark 6

To serve two, you can easily halve the quantities given or, as the fishburgers freeze well, you could make the full quantity given and freeze the extra fishburgers at step 4 (before they are cooked in the oven). Defrost fully at room temperature and then proceed from step 4.

450 g (1 lb) filleted whiting or other white fish
3–4 parsley stalks
1 slice lemon
300 ml (10 fl oz) Fish Stock (page 69) or water
salt and white pepper
1 large tomato
1 onion
2 tablespoons low-fat fromage frais or natural yogurt
2 tablespoons flour
1 quantity Tomato Sauce (page 235), to serve

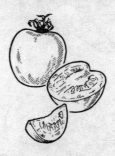

1. Skin the fish or ask your fishmonger to do this for you. Place in a frying-pan with the parsley stalks, slice of lemon and the fish stock or water. Season lightly with salt and white pepper. Cover with a lid and bring to the boil then simmer gently for 5–6 minutes. Remove the fish from the pan and drain well.

2. Remove the skin (page 246) and seeds from the tomato and chop the flesh. Peel and grate the onion.

3. Flake the fish and mix with the tomato, onion and fromage frais or yogurt. Add sufficient flour to bind the mixture then season well with salt and white pepper.

4. Form into four burger shapes and place on a non-stick baking sheet. Cook in a preheated oven at 200°C, 400°F, Gas Mark 6 for about 15 minutes until lightly browned.

5. Serve hot with Tomato Sauce.

MICROWAVE
The fish could be poached in a microwave.

SUGGESTED VEGETABLES
Oven Sauté Potatoes (page 196) or new potatoes.
Peas, beans, mange-tout, broccoli or carrots.

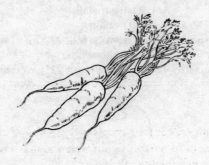

SMOKY FISH AND VEGETABLE PIE

Serves 4–5
Cooking time 25–35 minutes
Oven 200°C, 400°F, Gas Mark 6

This is an ideal family dish because it can be prepared in advance and cooked in the oven when required. It can also be frozen but without the prawns.

450–750 g (1–1½ lb) old potatoes
300 ml (10 fl oz) skimmed milk
450–750 g (1–1½ lb) smoked haddock fillets
100 g (4 oz) white button mushrooms
1 small onion
2 bay leaves
6 black peppercorns
3–4 parsley stalks
3–4 tomatoes
1 tablespoon cornflour
salt and white pepper
100 g (4 oz) cooked peas
100 g (4 oz) canned or frozen sweetcorn
100 g (4 oz) peeled prawns, optional

1. Peel the potatoes, cut into even-sized pieces and cook in boiling, salted water until tender. Drain well and mash with 2 tablespoons of milk until they are fluffy.
2. In the meantime, remove the skin and any bones from the fish and trim, clean and slice the mushrooms. Peel and slice the onion.
3. Place the fish in a frying-pan. Add the remainder of the milk, the mushrooms, onion, bay leaves, peppercorns and parsley stalks. Bring to the boil, cover and simmer gently for 5–8 minutes until the fish is tender.
4. Remove the fish and mushrooms from the pan, reserving the milk. Flake the fish coarsely. Skin (page 246) and slice the tomatoes.

---

5. Strain the milk and make up to 300 ml (10 fl oz) with water. Heat the milk in a pan. Mix the cornflour with a little water. Pour some of the hot milk over and mix well. Return to the pan and bring to the boil, stirring all the time, and cook for 1–2 minutes. Season to taste, taking care not to add too much salt as the milk will be slightly salty from the fish.

6. Mix the fish, mushrooms, peas and sweetcorn into the sauce. Add the prawns if they are to be used. Pour into a 1 litre (1¾ pint) pie dish. Place the sliced tomatoes over the fish. Season lightly and cover with the mashed potatoes. Cook in a preheated oven at 200°C, 400°F, Gas Mark 6 for 20–25 minutes. Serve hot.

MICROWAVE
Potatoes, fish and completed pie can all be cooked in a microwave but place the completed dish under a hot grill for a few minutes to brown before serving.

SUGGESTED VEGETABLES
Any green vegetable or carrots.

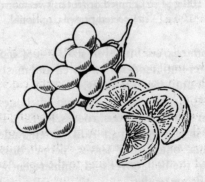

SMOKED MACKEREL WITH PASTA

Serves 4
Cooking time 20–25 minutes

This dish can also be made with tinned mackerel or tuna (buy the ones canned in brine) or with smoked haddock. The smoked haddock will need to be cooked before starting the recipe. A few shelled prawns can also be added to tuna or smoked haddock. Any pasta shape can be used but conchiglie (shells), fusilli (twists) or farfalle (butterfly twists) look most attractive. Consult the packet for cooking times.

450 g (1 lb) smoked mackerel fillets
1 onion
300 ml (10 fl oz) cider or Fish Stock (page 69)
2 tablespoons tomato purée
salt and white pepper
1 teaspoon arrowroot
3 tablespoons low-fat fromage frais or 75 g (3 oz) quark or
other low-fat soft cheese
225 g (8 oz) pasta of choice
1 tablespoon chopped fresh basil or parsley
a few fresh basil leaves or sprigs of parsley, to garnish

1. Skin the smoked mackerel fillets and remove any bones. Flake into reasonably sized pieces.
2. Peel and chop the onion and cook in the cider or fish stock until it is tender.
3. Pour the liquid into a measuring jug, measure it and make up to 300 ml (10 fl oz) with more cider, fish stock or water. Stir in the tomato purée and season to taste with salt and white pepper. Place the liquid in a pan and bring to the boil. Mix the arrow-root with a little water and pour into the pan. Bring to the boil, stirring all the time. Whisk the fromage frais, quark or other low-fat soft cheese into the sauce and stir in the flaked mackerel. Heat through without boiling. Check the seasoning.

---

4. In the meantime, cook the pasta in boiling, salted water. It will take about 10–12 minutes depending on the type used.

5. When the pasta is cooked, drain well and stir into the hot fish mixture with the chopped basil or parsley. Pile into a hot serving dish and garnish with fresh basil leaves or parsley sprigs just before serving. Serve hot.

MICROWAVE

The sauce and pasta can be microwaved but it is just as easy to use conventional cooking methods. Do not microwave the sauce after the fromage frais or quark has been added or the sauce will curdle.

SUGGESTED VEGETABLES

A salad can be served with or after this dish.

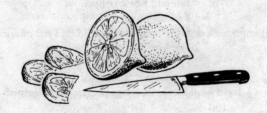

FLORENTINE FISH CROWN

Serves 5–6
Cooking time 30–40 minutes
Oven 200°C, 400°F, Gas Mark 6

If salmon fillet is not available (this is the whole side of salmon which has been filleted) use single pink trout fillets, or ask your fishmonger to fillet a tail piece of salmon and you can freeze the extra for another time. If you are using frozen spinach, do make certain that you use leaf spinach as chopped or puréed frozen spinach is too soft for this recipe. Maintenance dieters can cheat if they wish and use a can of Lobster Bisque with the prawns for the sauce.

6 x 75–100 g (3–4 oz) single plaice fillets
1 x 275–350 g (10–12 oz) piece filleted salmon
1 kg (2 lb) fresh spinach or 450 g (1 lb) frozen leaf spinach
100 g (4 oz) quark or other low-fat soft cheese
salt and white pepper
1 egg white
150 ml (5 fl oz) white wine or cider
150 ml (5 fl oz) skimmed milk
25 g (1 oz) cornflour
1–2 teaspoons tomato purée
100–150 g (4–6 oz) peeled prawns
a few whole prawns, to garnish, optional

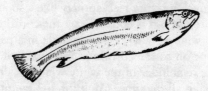

1. Skin the fillets of plaice and salmon or pink trout or ask your fishmonger to do this for you. Trim away any black membranes on the plaice. Cut the fillet of salmon into two down the seam where the backbone has been. Place the palm of your hand on

each piece of salmon and with a sharp knife cut each into three thin slices.

2. Lightly oil the inside of a non-stick 18 cm (7 inch) ring mould. Start with a slice of salmon and lay the salmon and plaice fillets alternately around the mould, taking care to cover the inside of the mould completely (see the photograph of this dish for the final effect). Make certain that the skin side of each fillet is uppermost (and will be covered by the filling) and have the tail ends in the centre of the mould. Cover and refrigerate while you proceed with the rest of the recipe.

3. Wash the fresh spinach well and remove any coarse stalks. Cook in boiling, salted water for 4–5 minutes. (If using frozen spinach , cook for 2–3 minutes.) Drain well in a colander and use a potato masher to press out as much water as possible so that the spinach is really dry.

4. Purée the spinach in a food processor or through a vegetable mill with half the quark or other low-fat soft cheese. Season well with salt and pepper. Whisk the egg white until it stands in stiff peaks and fold into the spinach mixture.

5. Wipe out any moisture in the bottom of the fish mould with kitchen paper and season lightly with salt and pepper. Pour the spinach into the mould and fold over any fish which is overlapping the inside or outside of the mould. Cover with aluminium foil and place in a roasting tin of boiling water. Cook in a preheated oven at 200°C, 400°F, Gas Mark 6 for 30–40 minutes until the spinach mixture feels springy like a sponge.

6. Just before the fish is cooked, mix the cornflour with a little of the white wine or cider. Place the milk in a pan and bring to the boil. Pour on to the cornflour and mix well. Return to the pan with the remainder of the white wine or cider and bring to the boil stirring all the time. Cook for 1–2 minutes. (If you boil the milk and white wine together, they will curdle.) Stir in sufficient tomato purée to give a warm pink colour then keep the sauce warm.

7. When the fish is cooked, whisk the remainder of the quark or other low-fat soft cheese into the sauce and then add the prawns.

Heat through without boiling. Turn the mould out on to a hot serving dish and pour a little of the sauce over. Serve the rest separately.

8. If you wish to garnish with whole prawns, peel the shell from the tail part only and place around the mound or in the centre. Serve hot.

MICROWAVE
The mould can be microwaved in a microwave-safe mould but make the sauce conventionally.

SUGGESTED VEGETABLES
New potatoes or Herby Mashed Potatoes (without the ham) (page 200). Peas, beans, mange-tout, broccoli, carrots, baby sweetcorn or Crispy Courgettes (page 206).

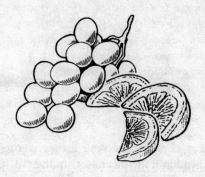

ST CLEMENT'S MACKEREL

Serves 4
Cooking time 30–35 minutes
Oven 160°C, 325°F, Gas Mark 3

4 mackerel approximately 225 g (8 oz) each
2 lemons
2 oranges
1 small onion
150 (5 fl oz) orange juice
50 g (2 oz) fresh breadcrumbs
1 tablespoon chopped parsley
1/4 teaspoon chopped dried rosemary
salt and black pepper
2–3 tablespoons orange marmalade

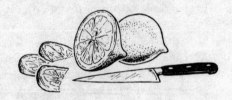

1. Fillet the mackerel or ask your fishmonger to do this for you. Cut off the head and the fins and trim the tail.
2. Grate the rind from 1 lemon and 1 orange. Squeeze the juice from the lemon. Cut the other lemon into thin slices (if you wish you can decorate it with a canelle knife – page 245 – first). Cut each slice in half and reserve for garnishing.
3. Cut the rind and pith from both oranges and cut out the segments from between the membranes. Chop the orange segments coarsely.
4. Peel and finely chop the onion. Place in a pan with the orange juice and cook gently for 6-7 minutes until the onion is slightly tender. Drain well, reserving the orange juice.

5. Mix the grated lemon and orange rinds and the lemon juice with the breadcrumbs, parsley, rosemary and the onion. Season well with salt and black pepper.

6. Season the inside of each mackerel. Divide the stuffing into four equal portions and place inside each fish. Place in a baking tin. Make the reserved orange juice up to 150 ml (5 fl oz) with water and pour around the fish. Spread a little marmalade over each one and bake in a preheated oven at 160°C, 325°F, Gas Mark 3 for 30–35 minutes until the fish is tender.

7. When the fish are cooked, transfer them to a hot serving dish and pour any juice in the pan over them. Keep hot and garnish with the reserved lemon slices just before serving.

MICROWAVE
The fish can be microwaved but only spread marmalade over 1¹/₂ minutes before the end of the cooking time. If necessary brown under a conventional grill.

SUGGESTED VEGETABLES
New potatoes, Oven Chips (page 195), or Oven Sauté Potatoes (page 196). Cauliflower, courgettes, peas. French or runner beans.

BROCHETTES OF FISH TANDOORI

Serves 4
Cooking time 10–15 minutes plus marinading time

750 g (1½ lb) filleted firm fish such as cod, monkfish,
rock salmon, swordfish or halibut
2 tablespoons tandoori powder
150 ml (5 fl oz) low-fat natural yogurt
1 tablespoon tomato purée
2 lemons or limes
1–2 Granny Smith apples
175–225 g (6–8 oz) rice or Savoury Brown Rice (page 158)
sprigs of fresh mint
lime pickle, optional

1. Cut the fish into large dice. Mix the tandoori powder with the yogurt, tomato purée and the juice of one of the lemons or limes. Toss the fish in the mixture until it is coated, then cover and leave to marinate in a refrigerator overnight or for 8 hours. Turn the fish occasionally if possible while it is marinating so that it is well coated.
2. Just before cooking the fish, cut the apples into thick slices and remove the cores. Cut each slice into four pieces. Cut the remaining lemon or lime into wedges.
3. Thread the fish and apple on to skewers and cook under a hot preheated grill or on a barbecue for about 5–7 minutes a side.
4. In the meantime, cook the rice or prepare the Savoury Brown Rice (page 158). When the rice is cooked, drain well and pile on a hot dish. Arrange the brochettes on top and garnish with lemon or lime wedges and sprigs of fresh mint. Serve hot with lime pickle if you wish.

MICROWAVE
Do not microwave.

SUGGESTED VEGETABLES
Green salad with Orange and Onion Salad (page 187).

FISH AND MUSHROOM TIMBALE

Serves 4
Cooking time 35–40 minutes plus 20 minutes for making stock
Oven 200°C, 400°F, Gas Mark 6

Fish stock is very easy to make. Ask your fishmonger for about 450 g (1 lb) fish trimmings, that is the skin and bones from any white fish except plaice (they make a bitter stock). Place the trimmings in a pan with 1 litre (1¾ pints) water. Add a peeled and sliced onion and carrot, a bay leaf and a few peppercorns and parsley stalks. Simmer gently for 20 minutes. Strain and use as required. Any excess can be frozen in small quantities. If you do not have any fish stock you can substitute fish stockcubes, which are now readily available, or vegetable stockcubes. You can also buy fresh ready-made fish stock in some supermarkets.

Do make certain to use small white mushrooms for the sauce; if you use larger ones they make the sauce grey.

browned breadcrumbs (page 71)
450 g (1 lb) cod, haddock or other white fish fillets
1 small onion
1 bay leaf
6 peppercorns
150 ml (5 fl oz) dry white wine or cider
150 ml (5 fl oz) fish stock (if you prefer, use 300 ml (10 fl oz) fish stock and omit the wine or cider)
50 g (2 oz) fresh white breadcrumbs
salt and white pepper
pinch nutmeg
2 egg whites
100 g (4 oz) white button mushrooms
225 g (7½ fl oz) skimmed milk
25 g (1 oz) cornflour

1. Lightly oil a non-stick 18 cm (7 inch) ring mould or deep sponge tin and dust well with the browned breadcrumbs.

---

2. Skin the fish or ask your fishmonger to do this for you. Peel and slice the onion. Place the onion, bay leaf and peppercorns in a pan and add the fish. Pour on the white wine or cider (if used) and the fish stock. Bring to the boil, cover then simmer gently for 7–8 minutes until the fish is tender. Remove the fish from the pan and flake it lightly with a fork. Reserve the fish liquor.

3. Strain and measure the fish liquor and make up to 300 ml (10 fl oz) with stock, wine, cider or water. Pour half into a pan (reserve the rest) and bring to the boil. Add the white breadcrumbs and season well with salt, pepper and a pinch of nutmeg. Beat well until it thickens.

4. Place the breadcrumb mixture in a large bowl and lightly mix in the fish. Whisk the eggs whites until they stand in soft peaks. Fold into the fish in two to three batches.

5. Spoon the mixture lightly into the prepared mould. Place in a roasting tin of boiling water and cook in a preheated oven at 200°C, 400°F, Gas Mark 6 for 25–30 minutes or until the fish mixture feels firm like a sponge.

6. In the meantime, clean, trim and slice the mushrooms. Cook for 6–8 minutes in the remaining fish liquor. Mix the cornflour with a little of the milk and add to the pan with 150 ml (5 fl oz) milk. Bring to the boil, stirring all the time, and cook for 2–3 minutes. Check the seasoning and, if the sauce is too thick, add more milk to give a coating consistency. Keep hot.

7. When the mould is cooked turn it out on to a hot serving dish and leave for 30–40 seconds before removing the mould or tin. Fill the centre of the mould with sauce (or, if you have used a sponge tin, pour a little sauce over the top). Serve the rest of the sauce separately. Serve hot.

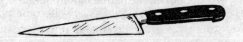

The fish, mould and sauce can be microwaved. Use a
microwave-safe mould.

SUGGESTED VEGETABLES
New or mashed potatoes (with skimmed milk or yogurt), Potato Quiche (page 191). Carrots, french or runner beans, peas or
broccoli.

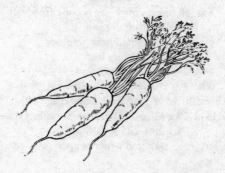

BROWNED BREADCRUMBS

To make browned breadcrumbs, make white or brown breadcrumbs in the usual way, then place them in a thin layer in a large
roasting tin. Bake them in a moderate oven until they are lightly
browned. You can often put them into an oven when you are
baking something else. Any temperature between 160°C, 325°F,
Gas Mark 3 to 200°C, 400°F, Gas Mark 6 can be used but watch
them carefully at the higher temperature so that they do not over-
brown. Shake the tin occasionally so that they are evenly
coloured. Place in a food processor to break down the breadcrumbs but don't overprocess or they will become powdery. If
you wish you can then sieve them to take out the coarser pieces.
Return these to the food processor until they are fine. These
breadcrumbs will keep for several months in an airtight container in a cupboard or in the deep freeze.

BRAISED TROUT

Serves 4–6
Cooking time 35–40 minutes
Oven 200°C, 400°F, Gas Mark 6

2 leeks
4 carrots
8 small onions (pickling onions are ideal)
4 small turnips
12–16 small new potatoes
1 bay leaf
5–6 peppercorns
3–4 parsley stalks
600 ml (1 pint) Fish Stock (page 69)
1 x 1.25–1.5 kg (2¹/₂–3 lb) salmon trout or salmon, or
4 x 200–225 g (7–8 oz) trout
salt and white pepper

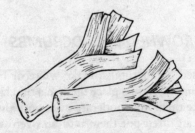

1. Wash and peel the leeks, carrots, onions and turnips. The potatoes can be scraped or the skins left on if you wish. Cut the leeks into two lengthways. Cut the carrots into four lengthways, and the turnips into quarters. Place in a pan with the bay leaf, peppercorns and parsley stalks. Pour in the fish stock, cover, bring to the boil and simmer for about 15 minutes until the vegetables are almost tender.
2. In the meantime, scale the fish, cut off the fins and trim the tail. Season well inside and out with salt and pepper.

3. When the vegetables are ready, pour them with the stock and the flavourings into a large dish or roasting tin and place the fish on top. Cover with a lid or aluminium foil and cook in a pre-heated oven at 200°C, 400°F, Gas Mark 6. A salmon trout or salmon will take about 30 minutes. Individual fish will take 15–20 minutes. To test if the fish is cooked, press it gently with a finger and the flakes under the skin should give slightly. Remove the peppercorns, bay leaf and parsley stalks.

4. To serve, place the fish on a large serving dish and arrange the vegetables around. Serve hot.

MICROWAVE

The vegetables and the trout could be microwaved but a larger fish would have to be cooked in the oven because of its size.

SUGGESTED VEGETABLES

This dish is a complete meal but if you wish you could serve a fresh summer vegetable such as peas, broccoli, french or runner beans.

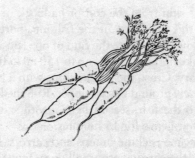

LEMONY COD

Serves 4
Cooking time 20–25 minutes

550–750 g (1¹/₄-1¹/₂ lb) cod or haddock fillet
2 lemons
extra lemon juice if required
salt
6–8 peppercorns
2–3 small onions
4–6 medium carrots
225 g (8 oz) mushrooms
300 ml (10 fl oz) Fish Stock (page 69) or vegetable stock
1 bay leaf
3–4 parsley stalks
4 tomatoes
1 teaspoon arrowroot
2 tablespoons low-fat fromage frais or low-fat natural yogurt
1 tablespoon chopped chives or chervil, to garnish

1. Remove the skin from the cod or haddock or ask your fish-monger to do this for you. Cut the fish into portions and place them in a shallow dish. Grate the rind of one lemon and the juice from both. Make the lemon juice up to 150 ml (5 fl oz) with extra juice, if necessary. Crush the peppercorns with a pestle and mortar or use coarsely ground black pepper. Rub the lemon rind and the pepper into the fish, season lightly with salt and pour the lemon juice over. Leave for 15 minutes.
2. In the meantime peel the onions and carrots. Finely slice the onions and cut the carrots into small dice. Trim, clean and slice the mushrooms.
3. Place the onions and carrots with the stock, bay leaf and parsley stalks in a frying-pan. Bring to the boil, cover and simmer gently for 5–6 minutes until the vegetables are almost tender. Add the mushrooms and cook for a further 2–3 minutes.
4. Meanwhile, skin (page 246), de-seed and coarsely chop the

tomatoes and stir them into the vegetables. Place the fish and the lemon juice on top, cover and cook gently for 8–10 minutes until the fish is cooked.

5. Transfer the vegetables to a hot dish and arrange the fish on top. Discard the bay leaf and parsley stalks. Mix the arrowroot with a little water and pour into the cooking liquor in the pan. Bring to the boil, stirring all the time. Stir in the fromage frais or yogurt, check the seasoning and pour the sauce over the fish and vegetables. Sprinkle with chopped chives or chervil just before serving. Serve hot.

MICROWAVE
Vegetables and fish can be microwaved but make the sauce in the conventional way.

SUGGESTED VEGETABLES
New potatoes, Oven Sauté Potatoes (page 196) or Herby Mashed Potatoes (page 200). No other vegetables are necessary but if you wish you can serve peas, beans, courgettes or broccoli.

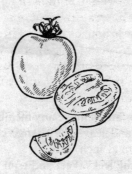

SCALLOPS AND MONKFISH WITH A VEGETABLE TAGLIATELLE

Serves 6–8 as a starter, 4 as a main course
Cooking time 15–20 minutes

If you prefer, use halibut or other firm white fish instead of the monkfish. You may also omit the scallops and increase the amount of white fish accordingly.

8 large scallops
225–350 g (8–12 oz) monkfish
2 medium leeks
2 long carrots
2 long courgettes
1–2 limes
150 ml (5 fl oz) Fish Stock (page 69)
150 ml (5 fl oz) white wine or white vermouth
2 tablespoons low-fat fromage frais or low-fat natural yogurt
pinch sugar (optional)
1/4–1/2 teaspoon curry powder
salt and white pepper

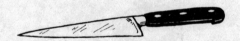

1. Wash the scallops and remove any membranes. Cut the white flesh into 2 pieces and leave the orange coral whole. Cut the monkfish into 2.5 cm (1 inch) dice.
2. Wash and trim the leeks. Peel and trim the carrots and trim the courgettes. Cut the leeks in half lengthways. With a mandolin or potato peeler, cut the carrots and courgettes into wafer-thin slices, down the length. Cut all the vegetables into 1 cm (1/2 inch) strips. Cut the limes into wedges.

3. Cook the leeks in the fish stock and white wine or vermouth for 1–2 minutes until almost tender. Add the carrots, bring back to the boil and cook for a further minute. Add the courgettes and cook for another minute. The vegetables should still have a 'bite' to them when they are cooked. Drain, returning the stock and wine to the pan. Cover the tagliatelle of vegetables and keep hot.

4. Poach the monkfish in the stock for 2–3 minutes then add the scallops and cook for a further minute. Take care not to over-cook the scallops or they will become tough. Remove from the stock, cover and keep warm.

5. Boil the stock until it has reduced to about 6-8 tablespoons. Remove from the heat. Stir in the fromage frais or yogurt and a pinch of sugar, if desired. Add sufficient curry powder to give just a hint of curry. Taste and season lightly with salt and pepper (extra seasoning may not be necessary if a fish stockcube has been used). Return to the heat and heat through without boiling.

6. Place the vegetables on a hot serving dish or individual dishes. Arrange the fish to one side of the plate or in the centre of the vegetables. Pour the sauce over the vegetables. Garnish the plate with wedges of lime and serve immediately.

MICROWAVE
Do not microwave.

SUGGESTED VEGETABLES
New potatoes. French beans, peas or mange-tout.

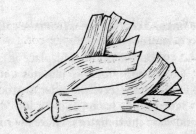

SAVOURY STUFFED CUTLETS

Serves 4
Cooking time 20–25 minutes
Oven 160°C, 325°F, Gas Mark 3

4 x 175–225 g (6–8 oz) cod, haddock or hake cutlets
1 small onion
150 ml (5 fl oz) cider or Fish Stock (page 69) or vegetable stock
2 rashers lean back bacon
2 tomatoes
1 lemon
2–3 tablespoons fresh breadcrumbs
1/2 teaspoon Herbes de Provence or herbs of choice
salt and black pepper
1 tablespoon chopped parsley, to garnish

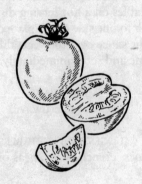

1. Remove the fins and central bones from the cutlets. Wash well and place in an ovenproof dish.
2. Peel and finely chop the onion and place in a pan with the cider or stock. Cook gently for 6–7 minutes until the onion is almost tender. Drain and reserve the cider or stock.
3. Remove any fat from the bacon and cut into dice. Skin (page 246), de-seed and chop the tomatoes. Grate the rind and squeeze the juice from the lemon.

4. Mix the breadcrumbs with the onion, bacon, tomatoes, grated lemon rind, lemon juice and the herbs. Season well with salt and black pepper and place an equal portion of the stuffing into the middle of each cutlet. Season the fish lightly. Make the reserved cider or stock up to 150 ml (5 fl oz) with more cider, stock or water and pour around the fish. Cover with a lid or aluminium foil and cook in a preheated oven at 160°C, 325°F, Gas Mark 3 for 20–25 minutes.

5. When the cutlets are cooked, transfer them to a hot serving dish. Cover and keep hot. Sprinkle chopped parsley over just before serving.

MICROWAVE
Can be microwaved.

SUGGESTED VEGETABLES
New potatoes, Oven Sauté Potatoes (page 196) or
mashed potatoes. Peas, beans, broccoli or
Crispy Courgettes (page 206).

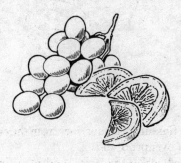

Poultry and Game

Chicken is so popular on the Hip and Thigh Diet but do you ever sit back and wonder how to give it a 'new look'? If so, I hope that this chapter will be the answer to your problems. Chicken Cicelia (page 83) with an interesting sauce of mushrooms and peppers, Chicken with a Barbecue Sauce (page 93), tangy and tasty for outdoor barbecues or suppers round the fire in winter or the delicious but different Chicken with Prawns (page 115) will all soon become family favourites.

Do try also the game recipes such as Venison with Blackcurrants (page 103), Pheasant with Orange (page 109) or Guinea Fowl with Lentils (page 111). They are all lean meats and ideal for this diet.

Buffet parties have not been forgotten. Learn how to bone and stuff a chicken (pages 85–89) – the finished dish will be well worth it. The Chicken and Mango Salad (95) not only looks attractive but tastes scrumptious with a hint of curry to complement the mango.

Microwave tips will again help you if you wish to use this method of cooking.

Poultry and Game

Ⓥ suitable for vegetarians
Ⓑ budget-conscious recipe
Ⓠ quick to prepare and cook

CHICKEN CICELIA

Serves 4
Cooking time 40–45 minutes
Oven 190°C, 375°F, Gas Mark 5

2 onions
100 g (4 oz) mushrooms
1/2 small green pepper
225 ml (7½ fl oz) chicken stock
4 teaspoons tomato purée
225 ml (7½ fl oz) white wine or cider
salt and black pepper
4 chicken breasts or 8 chicken thighs
2 teaspoons cornflour

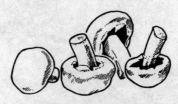

1. Peel the onions and chop coarsely. Clean and trim the mushrooms. Remove the stalk, seeds and pith from the pepper and cut into large pieces. Purée the onions, mushrooms and pepper in a food processor or liquidizer with 150 ml (5 fl oz) chicken stock. When the mixture is smooth add 150 ml (5 fl oz) white wine or cider and 2 teaspoons tomato purée. Season to taste with salt and black pepper.
2. Remove the skin from the chicken breasts or thighs and place them in an ovenproof dish. Pour the sauce over, cover with a lid and cook in a preheated oven at 190°C, 375°F, Gas Mark 5 for 40–45 minutes or until the chicken is tender.
3. When the chicken is cooked place it on a hot serving dish, cover and keep hot.
4. Transfer the sauce to a pan and add the remaining 75 ml (2½ fl oz) white wine or cider and the remaining 2 teaspoons tomato

---

purée. Bring to the boil. Mix the cornflour with the rest of the chicken stock and add to the pan. Bring to the boil again and boil for about 2 minutes, stirring all the time. Check the seasoning and adjust if necessary.

5. Pour the sauce over the chicken just before serving. Serve hot.

MICROWAVE
Can be microwaved.

SUGGESTED VEGETABLES
New potatoes, cauliflower, broccoli, carrots, peas, beans, sweetcorn kernels or baby sweetcorn.

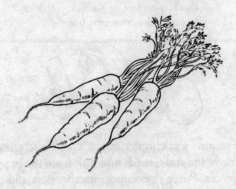

PARTY CHICKEN

This is a boned chicken and these are usually stuffed with a sausagemeat or other high-fat filling. This one is stuffed with chicken and ham and so is ideal for the Hip and Thigh Dieter. It makes a very special party dish and can easily be prepared in advance and stored in the deep freeze for up to 3 months. Allow 24 hours at a cool room temperature for it to defrost. Once it has defrosted refrigerate until required. If you wish to coat the chicken with aspic do this after it has defrosted completely.

Serves 8–10
Cooking time 2–2¼ hours
Oven 180°C, 350°F, Gas Mark 4

1 x 1.75 kg (3½ lb) chicken
3 x 100 g (4 oz) chicken breasts
4 thin slices Parma ham (page 37) or thin gammon rashers
4 chicken thighs
175 g (6 oz) lean ham or gammon steak
1 medium onion
1 teaspoon mixed herbs
1 tablespoon chopped parsley
75 g (3 oz) fresh white breadcrumbs
2 egg whites
2 tablespoons brandy
salt and black pepper

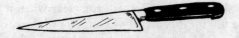

1. Bone the chicken (see page 87) or ask your butcher to do this for you. Remove the wing and thigh bones if this has not already been done. Tuck the flaps back inside the chicken. Leave the drumstick bones in place. Spread the boned chicken, flesh side up, on a board.

2. Under each breast you will find a long, pointed piece of flesh which can easily be detached. These are called the fillets. Remove these from the breasts on the boned chicken and from the extra breasts. Place these at the sides, centre and base of the breasts on the boned chicken so that you have an even layer of white meat.

3. Remove any fat from the Parma ham or thin gammon rashers. Place two of them over the chicken. Wrap the extra chicken breasts in the other slices of Parma ham or gammon.

4. Cut the bones from the four chicken thighs and discard (or use for stock). Peel and slice the onion. Finely chop the flesh from these thighs with the ham and onion in a food processor or pass through a mincer 2–3 times. Add the mixed herbs, parsley and breadcrumbs. Mix well. Lightly whisk the egg whites and work these into the mixture with the brandy. Season well with salt and black pepper. You will require about 1 teaspoon of salt. If you wish you can dry-fry a little of the mixture in a hot frying-pan to enable you to check the seasoning.

5. Spread a layer of the stuffing over the boned chicken. Place the breasts which have been wrapped in Parma ham or gammon rashers in the centre and cover with the remainder of the stuffing. Fold the sides over and sew up with a needle and strong white thread. Truss the legs with string to give a good shape to the chicken.

6. Lightly oil the base of a non-stick roasting tin. Place the chicken in the tin, cover with foil and roast in a preheated oven at 180°C, 350°F, Gas Mark 4 for 2–2¼ hours. To check that the bird is cooked, prick through the thighs to the centre of the bird with a fine skewer. The juices will run clear when it is cooked. Remove the foil for the last 30–40 minutes of the cooking time.

7. Cool thoroughly, then refrigerate or store in the deep freeze until required.

8. Remove the trussing strings and sewing thread from the bird and, if you wish, decorate it and coat it with aspic. Otherwise, slice the bird and place on a bed of lettuce to serve.

HOW TO BONE A CHICKEN

1 Trim the leg ends from the end of each drumstick. Cut off the wing tips and the first joint from each wing. Cut off the 'parson's nose'.

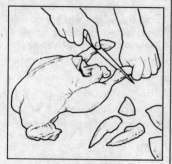

2 Remove the wishbone by scraping the front of each 'spur' of the wishbone with a small knife to expose the bone.

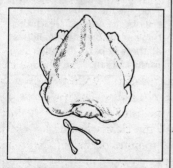

Run a finger and thumb along the bone to free it completely of flesh and with a finger break through the sinew holding the top of the bone to the carcass. Finally, with a sharp knife cut down each side of the wishbone at the base and pull it free from the carcass.

3 Turn the bird over and lay it breast down on a board. With a small, sharp knife slit the skin along the length of the backbone and with the knife scrape the flesh away from the carcass.

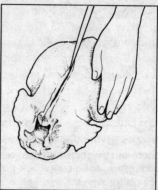

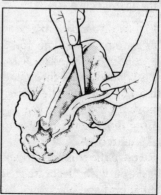

continued

---

4 When the thigh joint is exposed, press it outwards to break the joint. Cut through the joint, taking care not to cut through the skin.

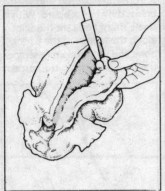

5 Scrape the flesh from each thigh and cut through the joint between the thigh and the drumstick, again taking care not to cut through the skin. Leave the drumstick in place.

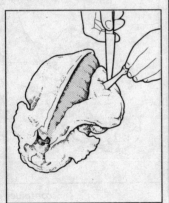

6 Scrape the flesh off the lower part of the ribcage and the shoulder bone. This is the flat bone that lies against the ribcage and is joined at the base to the wing joint. Continue easing the breast away from the carcass until the wing bones are exposed and remove the bones in the same way as the thigh bones.

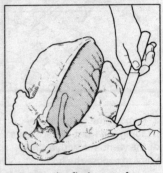

7 Scrape the flesh away from the ribcage until you reach the ridge of the breastbone. Repeat all these steps on the other side of the chicken.

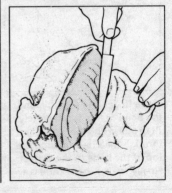

8 Taking great care not to break the skin, pull and scrape the breastbone away from the flesh. You will find that the skin of the bird is very close to the ridge of the breastbone so have the blade of the knife towards the bone all the time. If you are unfortunate enough to cut the skin, sew it up with a needle and strong white thread.

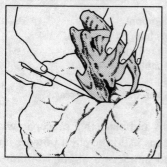

9 Tuck the skin and flesh from the wings inside the bird and when sewing it up after stuffing, secure with one or two stitches.

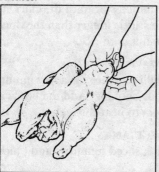

10 The bird is now ready to stuff. Use the carcass, the trimmings (free from all fat) and the bones from the extra thighs used in the stuffing (page 86) to make stock. Allow the stock to cool before use and skim all fat from the surface.

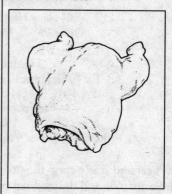

CHILLI CHICKEN

Chilli powder is available in mild or hot varieties. Chilli dishes are intended to be hot but if you prefer a mild one use the mild variety. Unless you are sure you like it hot, add 1 teaspoon to start with then gradually add more until it is as hot as you like.

Serves 4
Cooking time 35–40 minutes
Oven 200°C, 400°F, Gas Mark 6

2 medium onions
1 x 400 g (14 oz) can chopped tomatoes
1 x 400 g (14 oz) can red kidney beans
1–4 teaspoons chilli powder
salt
8 chicken thighs or 4 chicken quarters or breasts

1. Peel and finely chop the onions and place in a saucepan with the tomatoes and drained red beans. Add the chilli powder and salt to taste. Bring to the boil and simmer for about 10 minutes until the onions are tender.
2. In the meantime remove the skin from the chicken thighs or quarters and place them in an ovenproof casserole dish.
3. Pour the sauce over then cook in a preheated oven at 200°C, 400°F, Gas Mark 6 for about 30 minutes or until the chicken is tender. Chicken quarters will take a little longer than the thighs.
4. Check the seasoning and serve hot with rice.

MICROWAVE
Cook the onion, tomatoes and chilli together for a few minutes, then add the chicken and continue cooking. Add the beans at the end in time for them to heat through.

SUGGESTED VEGETABLES
Brown or white rice. Green salad, sliced tomatoes and onion rings.

CHICKEN AND TOMATO BAKE

Serves 4
Cooking time 45–50 minutes
Oven 200°C, 400°F, Gas Mark 6

2 medium onions
2 large carrots
2 sticks celery
450–550 g (1–1¼ lb) old potatoes
4 chicken breasts or quarters, or 8 chicken thighs
1 x 400 g (14 oz) can chopped tomatoes
150 ml (5 fl oz) cider or chicken stock
1 tablespoon tomato purée
1 bay leaf
salt and black pepper
chopped fresh coriander or parsley, to garnish

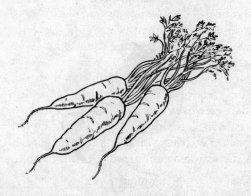

1. Peel the onions and carrots and trim and wash the celery.
Chop these vegetables into small dice. Peel and thinly slice the
potatoes.
2. Remove the skin and any fat from the chicken and place in an
ovenproof dish with the onion, carrot and celery. Pour over the
chopped tomatoes, cider or stock and the tomato purée. Add the
bay leaf and season to taste with salt and black pepper.

---

3. Cover with the sliced potatoes and season them lightly with salt. Cover with a lid and bake in a preheated oven at 200°C, 400°F, Gas Mark 6 for 45–50 minutes or until the vegetables and chicken are tender. Press the potatoes down into the stock once or twice while the dish is cooking so that they do not dry out. Remove the lid for the last 10 minutes or so of cooking time to allow the potatoes to brown on the top.

4. Sprinkle chopped coriander or parsley over the top just before serving.

MICROWAVE
This dish can be microwaved but brown finished dish under a hot grill.

SUGGESTED VEGETABLES
Cabbage, broccoli, green peas or beans, Brussels sprouts or cauliflower.

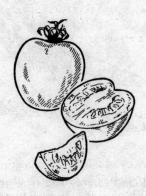

CHICKEN WITH BARBECUE SAUCE

If you wish to make this recipe for two people, you can either make the full quantity of sauce and freeze the surplus, or you can halve the recipe. In either case use two-thirds of the orange juice and cider in the full recipe when completing the dish.

Serves 4
Cooking time 20–40 minutes
Oven 190°C, 375°F, Gas Mark 5

2 tablespoons soy sauce
1 tablespoon Worcestershire sauce
1 tablespoon wine vinegar
2 tablespoons tomato ketchup
2 tablespoons clear honey
2 tablespoons orange marmalade or apricot jam
1 teaspoon French mustard
4 chicken breasts or portions
150 ml (5 fl oz) orange juice
150 ml (5 fl oz) cider
extra orange juice or cider, optional
1 teaspoon arrowroot
watercress, to garnish

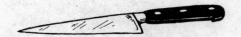

1. Mix together the soy sauce, Worcestershire sauce, wine vinegar, tomato ketchup, honey, marmalade or jam and the French mustard. Stir or whisk until the mustard has dissolved.
2. Remove the skin from the chicken breasts or portions. Place in a roasting tin and pour the sauce over. Cook in a preheated oven at 190°C, 375°F, Gas Mark 5. Chicken breasts will take 20–30 minutes and portions 30–45 minutes, depending on size. Spoon the sauce over the chicken 3–4 times while it is cooking.

As the sauce cooks it thickens and becomes syrupy and when you spoon it over the chicken it forms a complete coating. At this stage add half the orange juice and continue cooking without spooning the sauce over the chicken. If you are cooking chicken portions you may find it necessary to add more orange juice to the pan.

3. When the chicken is cooked, arrange it on a hot serving dish and keep hot. Pour the remainder of the orange juice and the cider into the roasting tin and stir well to incorporate all the caramelized sauce. Measure the liquid and make up to 300 ml (10 fl oz) with orange juice, cider or water. Pour into a pan and bring to the boil. Mix the arrowroot with a little water and add to the pan. Bring to the boil again, stirring all the time. Pour into a sauceboat to serve. Garnish the chicken with watercress just before serving and serve the sauce separately. Serve hot.

MICROWAVE
Not recommended as the sauce would caramelize too quickly.

SUGGESTED VEGETABLES
Herby Mashed Potatoes (page 200) or Dry Roast Potatoes (page 194). Oriental Cabbage (page 199), Brussels sprouts, spring greens, carrots or sweetcorn.

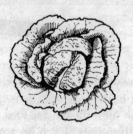

CHICKEN AND MANGO SALAD

Serves 6

175–225 g (6–8 oz) brown rice
1 x 1.5 kg (3½ lb) cold, cooked chicken
1 tablespoon juice of mango chutney
scant teaspoon curry powder or to taste
1 tablespoon soy sauce
1 teaspoon French mustard
300 ml (10 fl oz) low-fat fromage frais or low-fat natural yogurt
lemon juice or white wine vinegar to taste
salt and white pepper
1 ripe medium mango
5–6 spring onions
1 stick celery
1 orange
watercress, to garnish

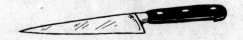

1. Cook the rice in boiling, salted water until tender. Drain then chill under cold running water and drain well again.
2. Remove the meat from the chicken carcass. Discard the skin and cut the meat into strips. Refrigerate until required.
3. Make the sauce by whisking the juice from the mango chutney with the curry powder, soy sauce and French mustard. When well mixed stir into the fromage frais or yogurt. Season to taste with a little lemon juice or vinegar, salt and pepper.
4. Peel the mango and remove the large seed from the middle. Cut about one-third of the flesh into neat slices and reserve for garnishing. Chop the remainder.
5. Trim and slice the spring onions and celery. Grate the rind from the orange and squeeze the juice.

---

6. Mix the rice with the spring onions, celery, grated rind of orange and about one-third of chopped mango. Stir in the orange juice and about 2–3 tablespoons of the dressing. Check the seasoning and adjust if necessary.

7. Mix the chicken with the remainder of the chopped mango and the dressing. Arrange the rice in a border on a flat dish and pile the chicken in the centre. Garnish with a circle of mango slices fanned out over the top of the chicken and with the watercress.

8. Cover with food wrap and refrigerate until required.

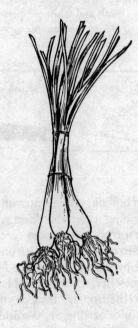

INDONESIAN CHICKEN

Serves 4–6
Cooking time approximately 1 hour 20 minutes

4 carrots
3 medium onions
2 sticks celery
1 leek
1 bay leaf
3–4 parsley stalks
6 peppercorns
1 x 1.5 kg (3½ lb) chicken
salt
100 g (4 oz) celeriac (page 198) or an extra celery stick
good pinch saffron or ¼ teaspoon turmeric
3–4 teaspoons curry powder or to taste
1 eating apple such as Granny Smith
1 banana
1 x 225 g (8 oz) can pineapple pieces in natural juice
225 g (8 oz) long-grain rice
chopped chives, to garnish

1. Peel the carrots and onions. Wash and trim the celery and leek. Reserve two carrots, one onion and one stick of celery and cut the remainder of the vegetables into large pieces. Tie the bay leaf and parsley stalks together with string and put into a large pan with the chopped vegetables and the peppercorns.
2. Remove any fat from the inside and place the chicken in the pan. Cover with cold water and season lightly with salt. Bring to the boil and simmer gently for about one hour until the chicken is tender.
3. Cut the remaining vegetables into medium-sized dice. If celeriac is used, place it in a bowl of cold water with a little lemon juice or vinegar to prevent it discolouring. Place the saffron (if used) into a small bowl and pour on two tablespoons of boiling water. Leave to infuse until required.

4. When the chicken is cooked remove it from the pan and measure 450 ml (15 fl oz) of the cooking stock into a pan. Add the vegetables, bring to the boil and cook for about 10 minutes until they are cooked but still have a 'bite'.
5. Remove the meat from the chicken. Discard the skin and bones and cut the flesh into strips.
6. When the vegetables are ready, stir in the curry powder and season to taste. Peel the apple and banana. Cut the banana into half down the length and then into slices. Core and dice the apple. Stir into the vegetables along with the chicken strips and pineapple pieces and heat through.
7. In the meantime, cook the rice in boiling, salted water until tender, drain well, return to the pan and stir in the saffron or turmeric. If saffron is used, it may be necessary to heat the rice until the liquid has evaporated. Stir in the chopped chives.
8. Pile the rice and chicken into separate dishes. Serve hot.

MICROWAVE
The chicken dish can be microwaved but it is possibly quicker to cook the rice conventionally at the same time as the chicken is in the microwave.

SUGGESTED VEGETABLES
This is a complete dish and requires no further vegetables.

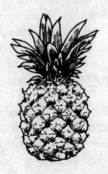

POULTRY AND GAME

SPICY YOGURT CHICKEN

Serves 4
Cooking time Grilling 20–30 minutes
Roasting 30–45 minutes, plus marinating overnight
Oven 200°C, 400°F, Gas Mark 6

Freshly ground spices give a better flavour but if whole pods or seeds are not available use powdered spices.

1 tablespoon green cardamom pods or
1 teaspoon ground cardamom
1 teaspoon coriander seeds
1 teaspoon cumin seeds
150 ml (5 fl oz) natural low-fat yogurt
1/4 teaspoon freshly ground nutmeg
1/4 teaspoon ground turmeric
1 tablespoon lemon juice
black pepper
4 chicken quarters or breasts
1 lemon, to garnish
watercress, to garnish

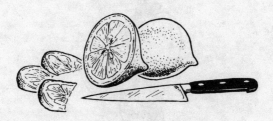

1. Shell the cardamom pods and remove the seeds – you need about 1 teaspoon of seeds. Grind the cardamom, coriander and cumin seeds or crush them with a pestle and mortar or in a strong bowl with the end of a rolling pin. Stir into the yogurt with the nutmeg, turmeric and lemon juice. Season with black pepper.

---

2. Skin the chicken pieces and place in a shallow dish. Pour the yogurt mixture over and leave to marinate in a refrigerator for 8 hours or overnight. Turn the chicken in the marinade 2–3 times if possible.

3. The chicken can be grilled or barbecued for 20–30 minutes or cooked in a preheated oven at 200°C, 400°F, Gas Mark 6 for 30–45 minutes. Both cooking times depend on the size and cut of chicken used.

4. Cut the lemon into wedges and when the chicken is cooked, arrange it on a hot serving dish and garnish with the lemon wedges and watercress just before serving. Serve hot.

MICROWAVE
Not advised as the yogurt will toughen in the microwave.

SUGGESTED VEGETABLES
Hot Vegetable Salad (page 197), Chicory and Apple Salad (page 186), Orange and Onion Salad (page 187) or green salad. Rice Pilaff (see Armenian Lamb Casserole, page 131) or Savoury Brown Rice (page 158).

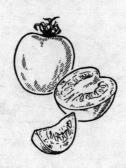

DUCK WITH ORIENTAL FRUIT SAUCE

Serves 4
Cooking time 18-20 or 35-45 minutes depending on cut used
Oven 220°C, 425°F, Gas Mark 7

Chicken breasts or quarters or lean pork or lamb chops can also be used in this recipe.

4 duck portions or breasts
2 tablespoons soy sauce
3 tablespoons clear honey
2 tablespoons dry sherry, cider or lemon juice
1 tablespoon white wine vinegar
1/4 teaspoon allspice
100 g (4 oz) kumquats or 2 small oranges
150 ml (5 fl oz) orange juice
150 ml (5 fl oz) duck or chicken stock
15 g (1/2 oz) fresh root ginger
8–10 fresh or canned lychees in natural juice
1 small extra orange
1–2 teaspoons arrowroot
watercress, to garnish

1. Remove the skin from the duck portions or breasts and place in a shallow dish.
2. Mix together 1 tablespoon soy sauce, 2 tablespoons honey, the sherry, cider or lemon juice, wine vinegar and the allspice. Pour over the duck and leave for 2–3 hours in the refrigerator. Spoon the marinade over the duck at frequent intervals.
3. Place the duck in a roasting tin and reserve the marinade. Cook in a preheated oven at 220°C, 425°F, Gas Mark 7. Duck breasts will take 18–20 minutes. Duck portions will take 35–45 minutes. Breasts need to be a little pink in the middle but duck leg portions are nicer if they are cooked right through. If the leg portions start to brown too much, turn the oven down to 190°C, 375°F, Gas Mark 5 and continue cooking until the juices run clear.

---

4. In the meantime, make the sauce. Cut each kumquat into 2–3 slices or cut the oranges into thick wedges and cut each wedge into 2–3 pieces. Place in a pan with the reserved marinade and the remainder of the soy sauce and honey. Add the orange juice and stock. Peel the ginger and grate 1 teaspoonful. (The remainder of the ginger can be frozen for another time.) Add the ginger to the pan, bring to the boil and simmer for 8–10 minutes. Peel the fresh lychees and cut fresh or canned lychees into quarters. Decorate the extra orange with a canelle knife (page 245) if you wish, or cut into thin slices. Cut each slice in half. Reserve for garnishing.

5. When the duck is cooked, arrange it on a hot serving dish, cover and keep hot. Mix the arrowroot with a little water and stir into the sauce. Bring to the boil again, stirring all the time. Add the lychees and heat through. Pour a little sauce over the duck and pour the rest into a sauceboat. Garnish the dish with the orange slices and watercress just before serving. Serve hot.

MICROWAVE
Best cooked conventionally.

SUGGESTED VEGETABLES
Oriental Cabbage (page 199), Farmer's-style Mange-tout (page 189), broccoli or french beans. Oven Sauté Potatoes (page 196) or Dry Roast Potatoes (page 194).

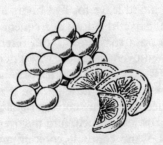

VENISON WITH BLACKCURRANTS

Venison is a very lean meat and casseroling venison is reasonably inexpensive and costs about the same as stewing beef. It has a delicious flavour which is enhanced by the blackcurrants. Do make certain that you serve venison piping hot as the fat in the flesh congeals at a higher temperature than other meats. This recipe is also delicious used with lean lamb or pork.

Serves 4–6
Cooking time 2¹/₂–3 hours, plus marinating overnight
Oven 160°C, 325°F, Gas Mark 3

1 large onion
1 large carrot
750 g (1¹/₂ lb) casseroling venison
12 peppercorns
1 bay leaf
300 ml (10 fl oz) red wine
300 ml (10 fl oz) beef stock
350 g (12 oz) blackcurrants, fresh or frozen
pinch sugar
salt and black pepper
2–3 teaspoons arrowroot
chopped parsley, to garnish

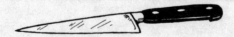

1. Peel and slice the onion and carrot. Trim the venison and remove any coarse sinews. Place the venison in a deep dish with the onion, carrot, peppercorns and bay leaf. Pour on the wine, cover and refrigerate overnight.
2. Remove the meat and vegetables separately from the marinade, drain well and reserve. Remove the bay leaf and peppercorns, reserve the bay leaf but discard the peppercorns. Reserve the marinade.

3. Place a frying-pan over the heat and dry-fry the well-drained meat a little at a time until it is well browned. Place in a flame-proof casserole with the onion and carrot, the red wine and bay leaf used for the marinade, the stock and the blackcurrants. Add a pinch of sugar and season to taste with salt and black pepper. Bring to the boil and place in a preheated oven at 160°C, 325°F, Gas Mark 3 for 2½–3 hours or until the meat is tender.

4. With a draining spoon remove the meat from the casserole and place in a hot serving dish. Cover and keep hot. Remove and discard the bay leaf. Lightly purée the sauce for a moment or two. The pips in the blackcurrants become gritty if they are over-puréed. Strain the sauce through a nylon sieve and make up to 600 ml (1 pint) with more red wine or stock if needed. Bring to the boil. Mix the arrowroot with a little water and add to the sauce. Bring to the boil again, stirring all the time. Pour over the meat and sprinkle chopped parsley over just before serving. Serve hot.

MICROWAVE
Venison could be microwaved on a simmer setting.

SUGGESTED VEGETABLES
Celeriac and Potato Purée (page 204) or new potatoes. Crispy Courgettes (page 206), Farmer's-style Mange-tout (page 189), Oriental Cabbage (page 199), broccoli, french beans or peas.

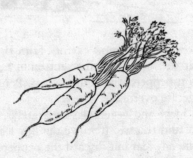

STUFFED TURKEY ESCALOPES

Serves 4
Cooking time 45–50 minutes
Oven 190°C, 375°F, Gas Mark 5

Thin pork escalopes can also be used in this recipe.

50 g (2 oz) lean ham
175 g (6 oz) button mushrooms
1 medium onion
2–3 tablespoons fresh white or brown breadcrumbs
grated rind of 1 lemon
1/2 teaspoon mixed herbs
2 tablespoons chopped parsley
1 egg white
salt and black pepper
4 x 100–175 g (4–6 oz) thin turkey escalopes
300 ml (10 fl oz) cider or chicken stock
1 tablespoon tomato purée
1 teaspoon arrowroot

1. Remove any fat from the ham and chop finely. Clean and trim the mushrooms. Chop 50 g (2 oz) of the mushrooms very finely. Halve or quarter the rest and reserve. Peel and grate the onion. Mix the ham, chopped mushrooms and onion with the breadcrumbs, lemon rind, mixed herbs and most of the parsley. Whisk the egg white until it is slightly frothy and mix well into the stuffing to bind it together. Season well with salt and black pepper.
2. Spread the turkey escalopes out on a board. Divide the stuffing equally and place a portion on each escalope. Fold the sides over to enclose the stuffing and roll up. Secure with cocktail sticks or tie with string.
3. Dry-fry the escalopes in a hot frying-pan until they are lightly browned. Place in a flameproof dish and pour on the cider or stock and stir in the tomato purée. Season to taste and cook in a preheated oven at 190°C, 375°F, Gas Mark 5 for 45–50 minutes

until they are tender. Add the reserved mushrooms 10–15 minutes before the end of the cooking time.

4. When the escalopes are cooked, place them in a hot serving dish, cover and keep hot. Mix the arrowroot with a little water. Add to the pan and bring to the boil, stirring all the time. Check the seasoning and pour over the escalopes. Sprinkle chopped parsley over just before serving.

MICROWAVE
Can be microwaved.

SUGGESTED VEGETABLES
Herby Mashed Potatoes (page 200), new potatoes or Oven Sauté Potatoes (page 196). Farmer's Style Mange-tout (page 189), Celeriac Paysanne (page 198), Oriental Cabbage (page 199), or any green vegetable.

FREEZING
Can be deep frozen when cooked.

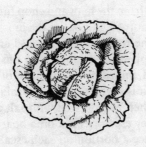

SWEET 'N' SOUR CHICKEN

Serves 4
Cooking time 40–45 minutes
Oven 180°C, 350°F, Gas Mark 4

8–10 chicken thighs (boneless ones are best)
2 teaspoons powdered ginger
1 red pepper
4 tomatoes
5 tablespoons white or red wine vinegar
3 tablespoons demerara sugar
2 tablespoons soy sauce
300 ml (10 fl oz) chicken stock
1 x 225 g (8 oz) can pineapple pieces in natural juice
1½ tablespoons cornflour
225 g (8 oz) long-grain white or brown rice

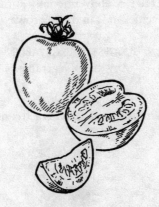

1. Remove the skin from the chicken thighs and also remove the bone if necessary. Cut each thigh into 4–5 pieces. Place in an ovenproof dish and sprinkle the ginger on to the chicken pieces and mix in well. Leave for at least 15 minutes.
2. Remove the stalk, pith and seeds from the red pepper and cut into strips. Skin (page 246) and quarter the tomatoes.

3. In a pan, mix together the vinegar, sugar, soy sauce, chicken stock and the juice from the canned pineapple. Bring to the boil. Mix the cornflour with a little water. Pour on some of the hot liquid and mix well. Return to the pan and bring to the boil again, stirring all the time.

4. Add the pepper, tomatoes and the pineapple pieces to the sauce and pour over the chicken. Cover with a lid and cook in a preheated oven at 180°C, 350°F, Gas Mark 4 for 40–45 minutes until the chicken is tender.

5. Meanwhile boil the rice in boiling, salted water until cooked. Drain well and make into a border on a hot serving dish. Pour the cooked chicken into the centre or, if you wish, you can serve the chicken and rice separately. Serve hot.

MICROWAVE
This dish can be cooked in the microwave but you may find it quicker to cook the rice conventionally at the same time as the chicken is in the microwave.

SUGGESTED VEGETABLES
Any green vegetable.

FREEZING
This dish is suitable for freezing.

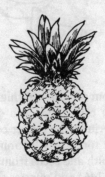

PHEASANT WITH ORANGE

Hen pheasants are smaller birds than cock pheasants and their flesh is slightly more tender. This recipe is excellent for older birds but in this case allow extra cooking time and cook at 160°C, 325°F, Gas Mark 3 until they are tender. It may also be necessary to add more stock to keep them moist while cooking.

Serves 4
Cooking time 1–1¼ hours
Oven 180°C 350°F, Gas Mark 4

1 pheasant
100 g (4 oz) mushrooms
3 medium onions
2 oranges
150 ml (5 fl oz) pheasant or chicken stock
150 ml (5 fl oz) orange juice
4 tablespoons dry sherry
salt and black pepper
1 teaspoon arrowroot
chopped parsley, to garnish

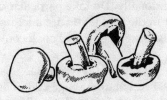

1. Cut the pheasant into four portions by cutting through the skin between the thigh and the body. Press the leg and thigh down on to the board and this will open and dislocate the joint. Cut through the joint with a sharp knife. Do the same on both sides. Remove and discard the scaly ends of the leg. Cut through the carcass along the breastbone and down through the backbone. Remove and discard the first two joints of the wing and cut off surplus breastbone and backbone with a pair of scissors.

2. Trim, clean and slice the mushrooms. Peel and chop the onions. Grate the rind from one orange then cut off the pith and cut out the segments from between the membranes. Cut each segment into 2–3 pieces. Slice the other orange thinly. If you wish you can decorate it with a canelle knife (page 245) first. Cut each slice in half and reserve.

3. Dry-fry the pieces of pheasant in a hot frying-pan until they are lightly coloured. Add the onions, grated orange rind, stock, orange juice and sherry. Bring to the boil then transfer to an ovenproof dish. Season to taste, cover and cook for 1–1¼ hours in a preheated oven at 180°C, 350°F, Gas Mark 4 or until the pheasant is tender. Add the orange segments and mushrooms about 15 minutes before the end of the cooking time.

4. When the pheasant is cooked, arrange it in a hot serving dish. Pour the sauce into a pan, mix the arrowroot with a little water and add to the pan. Bring to the boil, stirring all the time. Pour over the pheasant. Sprinkle chopped parsley over and garnish with the orange slices just before serving. Serve hot.

MICROWAVE
Young birds could be microwaved but I would prefer to cook older birds conventionally. Do take particular care that there is no lead shot left in the bird if you are microwaving it. If the bird is badly shot, play safe and cook conventionally.

SUGGESTED VEGETABLES
Herby Mashed Potatoes (page 200), Potato and Celeriac Purée (page 204) or Dry Roast Potatoes (page 194). Oriental Cabbage (page 199), Farmer's-style Mange-tout (page 189), french beans, broccoli, baby sweetcorn or courgettes.

FREEZING
Can be deep frozen when cooked.

GUINEA FOWL WITH LENTILS

Serves 4
Cooking time 1–1¼ hours
Oven 200°C, 400°F, Gas Mark 6

Not all brown or green lentils need to be soaked so consult the directions on the packet you use. If in doubt soak them first.

225 g (8 oz) brown lentils
2 large onions
1 bay leaf
3–4 parsley stalks
a small piece of celery
salt and black pepper
1 x 1.5 kg (3½ lb) guinea fowl
100 g (4 oz) ham steak without fat
300 ml (10 fl oz) chicken stock
1 tablespoon tomato purée
1 teaspoon arrowroot
watercress, to garnish

1. If necessary pour boiling water over the lentils and leave for 40–50 minutes. Peel the onions. Slice one onion. Finely chop the other and reserve. Tie the bay leaf, parsley stalks and celery together with string to make a bouquet garni. Drain the lentils and rinse then place in a large pan with the sliced onion and bouquet garni. Bring to the boil and simmer for 30–40 minutes or until tender. Season with salt and pepper just before the end of the cooking time.
2. Meanwhile place the guinea fowl in a roasting tin in a preheated oven at 200°C, 400°F, Gas Mark 6 for 1–1¼ hours or until the juices in the bird run clear.
3. When the lentils are cooked drain them well but leave enough cooking liquid to keep them moist. Remove the bouquet garni. Check the seasoning, cover and keep hot.

4. In the meantime make the sauce. Remove any fat from the ham and cut into small dice. Cook the reserved chopped onion in the stock until tender, then stir in the tomato purée. Mix the arrowroot with a little water and add to the pan. Bring to the boil again, stirring all the time. Stir in the ham, taste and season.

5. When the bird is cooked, remove the trussing strings and carve or joint it. Place the lentils on a hot serving dish. Arrange the sliced or jointed bird down the centre. Pour a little sauce over and serve the rest separately in a sauceboat. Garnish with watercress just before serving. Serve hot.

MICROWAVE

The guinea fowl could be microwaved but cook with the stock. Make the sauce conventionally, making up the quantity (if necessary) to the original amount. You may like to flash the bird under a hot grill to brown it once it is cooked.

SUGGESTED VEGETABLES

New potatoes or Dry Roast Potatoes (page 194). Farmer's-style Mange-tout (page 189), french or runner beans, carrots, Brussels sprouts or spinach.

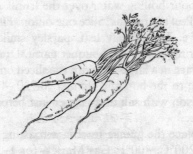

CHICKEN LIVERS WITH MIXED VEGETABLES

Serves 4
Cooking time 20–30 minutes

The selection of vegetables in this recipe give a colourful variety but you can use any selection. Peas, french beans or baby sweet corn could be substitutes for the mushrooms or mange-tout.

450g (1 lb) small new potatoes
175 g (6 oz) button onions
175 g (6 oz) small carrots
100 g (4 oz) button mushrooms
75 g (3 oz) mange-tout
3–4 small leeks
600 ml (1 pint) chicken or vegetable stock
salt and black pepper
1/2 teaspoon chopped thyme
450–550 g (1–11/4 lb) chicken livers
1 teaspoon arrowroot, optional
chopped parsley, to garnish

1. Scrape the potatoes, peel the onions and scrape or peel the carrots. Trim and clean the mushrooms, top and tail the mange-tout. Trim and wash the leeks. Cut the carrots and leeks into thick slices (unless the carrots are very small when they can be left whole).
2. Place the potatoes and onions in a pan with the stock. Bring to the boil and simmer for 7–10 minutes. Add the carrots and simmer for 5 minutes. Add the leeks and cook for another 5 minutes then add the mange-tout and mushrooms. Cook until all the vegetables are just tender. Drain, reserving the stock for soup (or if you wish you can thicken 300 ml (10 fl oz) of the stock with arrowroot to serve with the finished dish). Sprinkle the thyme over the vegetables and mix in lightly, cover and keep hot.

---

3. In the meantime, trim any sinews from the livers and cut out any yellowish green parts (this is where they have been stained by the gall-bladder and will be bitter to eat). Dry-fry the livers in a hot frying-pan until they are just pink in the middle.

4. Mix the livers and vegetables together and pile into a hot dish. Sprinkle chopped parsley over just before serving. Serve hot.

MICROWAVE
Vegetables could be microwaved but they are just as quick to cook conventionally.

SUGGESTED VEGETABLES
This is a complete dish, no other vegetables are necessary.

FREEZING
Not suitable for freezing but frozen livers can be bought and stored in the deep freeze until required. Thaw completely before use.

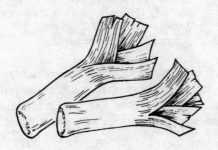

CHICKEN WITH PRAWNS

Serves 4
Cooking time 30–35 minutes
Oven 200°C, 400°F, Gas Mark 6

1 onion
150 ml (5 fl oz) Fish Stock (page 69)
150 ml (5 fl oz) white wine or cider
2–3 teaspoons tomato purée
4 boneless chicken breasts
salt and white pepper
2 tomatoes
1 teaspoon arrowroot
100–175 g (4–6 oz) peeled prawns
2 tablespoons low-fat fromage frais or low-fat natural yogurt
watercress, to garnish

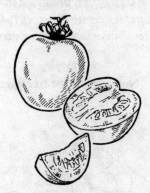

1. Peel and finely chop the onion and place in a pan with the fish stock and wine or cider. Bring to the boil and simmer for 8–10 minutes until almost tender. Stir in 2 teaspoons tomato purée.
2. Remove the skin from the chicken and place in an ovenproof dish. Pour over the stock and onion, cover and season lightly. Place in a preheated oven at 200°C, 400°F, Gas Mark 6 and cook for 20–25 minutes until the chicken is tender.

3. In the meantime, skin (page 246), de-seed and cut the tomatoes into small dice.

4. When the chicken is cooked, place it in a hot serving dish, cover and keep hot. Return the stock and wine to a pan and bring to the boil. Mix the arrowroot with a little water and add to the pan. Bring to the boil again, boiling all the time. Stir in the prawns, fromage frais or yogurt and the diced tomatoes. Check the seasoning and add a little more tomato purée if necessary to give a warm pink colour. Heat through gently without boiling. Pour the sauce and prawns over the chicken. Garnish with watercress just before serving. Serve hot.

MICROWAVE
The onion and chicken could be cooked in the microwave but make the sauce conventionally.

SUGGESTED VEGETABLES
New potatoes or Oven Sauté Potatoes (page 196). Spinach, courgettes, Brussels sprouts or green beans.

FREEZING
Not suitable for freezing.

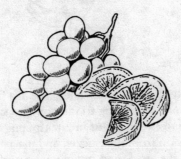

Meat

The more I experiment, the more dishes I find that are just as tasty when cooked without fat. Here you will find another selection of meat recipes, some new and some adaptations of old favourites, all without extra fat. Do try the Lamb and Red Bean Casserole (page 119), or enjoy the subtle spicy flavour of the Armenian Lamb Casserole (page 131), or the lovely flavour of the Beef Carbonnade (page 128) with the gravy made with beer. The Guinness Hot-pot (page 149) is ideal for wintry days and the Honeyed Pork with Tagliatelle (page 147) will soon become a favourite as it is so quick and easy to prepare.

All the recipes in this chapter can be eaten as part of the main meal of the day by Hip and Thigh Dieters and those on the Maintenance Diet alike, accompanied by a selection of vegetables and potatoes or rice. Hip and Thigh Dieters are reminded that they should eat red meat only twice a week.

Microwave tips have also been given again, in case you want to use this method of cooking.

Meat

Ⓥ suitable for vegetarians
Ⓑ budget-conscious recipe
Ⓠ quick to prepare and cook

LAMB AND RED BEAN CASSEROLE

Serves 4–5
Cooking time 1–1¹/₂ hours
Oven 180°C, 350°F, Gas Mark 4

550 g (1¹/₄ lb) lean lamb without bones
100 g (4 oz) lean bacon
2 medium onions
2 carrots
1 tablespoon flour
225 ml (7¹/₂ fl oz) lamb or chicken stock
300 ml (10 fl oz) red wine
1 x 400 g (14 oz) can red kidney beans
salt and black pepper
1 bay leaf
3–4 parsley stalks
small piece of celery

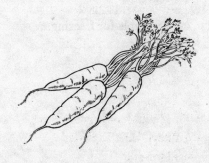

1. Trim any fat from the lamb and bacon. Cut the lamb into dice and the bacon into strips. Dry-fry the lamb in a hot frying-pan until golden brown (page 245).
2. Peel the onions and carrots. Finely chop the onions and slice the carrots.
3. Stir the flour into the meat and mix well, then add the stock and wine a little at a time, stirring well to prevent any lumps forming. Transfer to an ovenproof dish and add the bacon,

onions and carrots. Drain the beans and rinse under the cold tap. Add to the pan and season to taste. Tie the bay leaf, parsley stalks and celery together and add to the pan. Cover and cook in a pre-heated oven at 180°C, 350°F, Gas Mark 4 for 1–1½ hours until the meat is tender.

4. Remove the bay leaf, parsley stalks and celery. Check the seasoning. If you wish transfer to a hot serving dish or serve in the cooking dish.

MICROWAVE
Can be microwaved on a simmer setting but add beans just before cooking time is ended. It may be necessary to reduce the stock.

SUGGESTED VEGETABLES
Mashed potatoes (with skimmed milk or low-fat yogurt), new potatoes or rice. Any green vegetable.

FREEZING
Suitable for freezing.

APRICOT STUFFED LAMB

Serves 1.5 kg (3½ lb) leg serves 6–7
1.25 kg (2–2½ lb) half leg serves 4
Cooking time 30 minutes per 450 g (l lb) weighed after stuffing
Oven 180°C, 350°F, Gas Mark 4

This is an ideal family or party roast. If you find a whole leg is too big for you, buy a half leg. You will find the shank end is easier to stuff. Or, if you wish you can stuff a whole leg and, when it is tied, cut it into two and freeze half for another occasion. A shoulder of lamb can also be stuffed in this way but do make sure it is very lean and cut out all visible fat.

1.5 kg (3½ lb) leg of lamb
175 g (6 oz) ready-to-eat dried apricots
1 medium onion
2 oranges
75 g (3 oz) fresh white or brown breadcrumbs
1 teaspoon chopped fresh or dried rosemary
salt and black pepper
300 ml (10 fl oz) orange juice
½ teaspoon beef or vegetable extract
1–2 teaspoons arrowroot

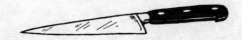

1. Remove the bone from the leg or ask your butcher to do this for you. Cut out any fat inside the leg but try not to cut through the skin.
2. Chop the apricots into moderate-sized pieces. Peel and finely chop the onion. Grate the rind and squeeze the juice of the oranges. Mix together the apricots, onion, breadcrumbs and rosemary with the grated rind of both oranges and the juice of

one orange. Reserve the juice from the other orange. Season well with salt and black pepper. Press the stuffing into the cavity in the lamb and skewer and tie up to make it secure.

3. Weigh the lamb and cook it in a preheated oven at 180°C, 350°F, Gas Mark 4 for 30 minutes per 450 g (1 lb). Add on another 15–20 minutes if you like your lamb well done.

4. When the lamb is cooked, remove it from the oven and keep hot.

5. Make the reserved orange juice up to 300 ml (10 fl oz) with the extra orange juice and pour into a pan. Stir in the beef or vegetable extract and bring to the boil. Mix the arrowroot with a little water, add to the pan and bring to the boil, stirring all the time. Season to taste, adding a little more beef or vegetable extract if you wish.

6. Slice the meat and stuffing and place on a hot serving dish. Pour a little sauce over and serve the rest separately. Serve hot.

MICROWAVE
Microwaving is not recommended.

SUGGESTED VEGETABLES
Dry Roast Potatoes (page 194) or creamed potatoes (with skimmed milk or low-fat natural yogurt). Spinach, cauliflower, Celeriac Paysanne (page 198), cabbage, peas or beans.

SPICED BEEF AND BEAN CASSEROLE

Serves 4
Cooking time 1¹/2–2¹/2 hours
Oven 180°C, 350°F, Gas Mark 4

This recipe, like several others in the book, has a Middle Eastern influence with its subtle use of spices. If you prefer a stronger flavour adjust the spices accordingly, especially the fresh grated ginger.

450–550 g (1–1¹/2 lb) lean chuck or bladebone steak
1 teaspoon ground coriander
¹/2 teaspoon powdered cumin
¹/4 teaspoon ground or fresh grated ginger
1 large onion
2 cloves garlic or 1 teaspoon garlic paste
1 red pepper
1 x 400 g (14 oz) can red kidney beans
300 ml (10 fl oz) beef stock or water
1 x 400 g (14 oz) can chopped tomatoes
2 tablespoon tomato purée
1–2 teaspoons Chinese chilli sauce or to taste
salt
chopped parsley, to garnish

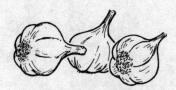

1. Remove any fat and cut the meat into 2.5 cm (1 inch) dice. Place a frying-pan over the heat and, when it is hot, dry-fry the meat (about one-third at a time) until it is well browned on all sides (page 245). Add the spices and cook for 2–3 minutes.

2. Meanwhile, peel the onion and garlic. Slice the onion and crush the garlic. Remove the stalk, pith and seeds from the pepper and cut into 1 cm (1/2 inch) dice. Drain and rinse the red beans.

3. Add the stock or water and the tomatoes to the pan and stir round very well to incorporate all the spices. Bring to the boil and pour into an ovenproof dish with the onion, garlic, red pepper, beans and the tomato purée. Add chilli sauce to taste and season with salt. Cover and cook in a preheated oven at 180°C, 350°F, Gas Mark 4 for 2–2½ hours until the meat is tender. Check the seasoning, adding more salt and/or chilli sauce if necessary.

4. Serve in the cooking dish or transfer to a hot serving dish. Sprinkle chopped parsley over the top just before serving. Serve hot.

MICROWAVE
This dish can be microwaved on a simmer setting. It may be necessary to reduce the stock.

SUGGESTED VEGETABLES
Creamed potato (with skimmed milk or
low-fat natural yogurt), jacket potatoes or rice.
Any green vegetable.

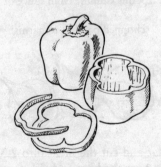

PORK AND PRUNES

Serves 4
Cooking time 25–30 minutes

1 large onion
8–10 ready-to-cook prunes
300 ml (10 fl oz) cider
450–550 g (1–1¼ lb) lean pork fillet
1 orange
1 extra orange, optional, to garnish
150 ml (5 fl oz) orange juice
1 tablespoon mango chutney
salt and black pepper
1 teaspoon arrowroot
chopped parsley, to garnish

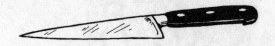

1. Peel and chop the onion and place in a pan with the prunes and cider. Bring to the boil and simmer for 10–12 minutes until the onion and prunes are tender. Remove the prunes, cover and keep hot, then boil the cider rapidly to reduce by one-third.
2. Trim away any fat on the pork and cut into large dice. Dry-fry in a hot frying-pan until browned all over and almost cooked through.
3. Grate the rind and squeeze the juice from the orange. If you wish you can slice an extra orange, cut each slice in half and reserve for garnishing. Measure the squeezed juice from the orange and make up to 150 ml (5 fl oz) with the extra orange juice. Mix the orange juice with the cider and pour on to the pork. Stir in the mango chutney and grated orange rind and season to taste with salt and black pepper. Simmer for 10–12 min-

utes until the pork is tender. Mix the arrowroot with a little water, add to the pan and bring to the boil, stirring all the time. 4. Pour into a hot serving dish and sprinkle chopped parsley over just before serving. Serve hot.

MICROWAVE
This can be microwaved on a simmer setting but I find it just as easy to use the method in the recipe.

SUGGESTED VEGETABLES
Rice, pasta, new or mashed potatoes (with skimmed milk or low-fat natural yogurt). Cabbage, Brussels sprouts, cauliflower, runner beans, peas or sweetcorn.

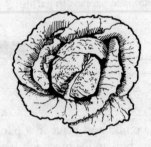

PROVENÇALE KIDNEYS

Serves 4
Cooking time 20–30 minutes

10–12 lamb's kidneys
450 g (1 lb) tomatoes
2 medium onions
2 cloves garlic or 1 teaspoon garlic paste
1 teaspoon chopped fresh basil or ½ teaspoon dried basil
225ml (7½ fl oz) red wine or beef stock
salt and black pepper
2 teaspoons flour

1. Skin the kidneys, cut in half and cut out the cores. Place in a bowl of cold, salted water and leave to soak for 20 minutes.
2. Skin (page 246) and de-seed the tomatoes. Remove the seeds and cut the flesh into dice. Peel the onions and garlic. Finely chop the onion and crush the garlic.
3. Place the tomatoes in a pan with the onions, garlic, basil and the red wine or beef stock. Season to taste and simmer gently until the onions are tender. If necessary add a little stock or water to give a coating consistency.
4. Drain the kidneys and dry well on kitchen paper. Dry-fry them in a hot frying-pan until they are well browned (page 245). Stir in the flour and mix well. Pour on the sauce and cook gently for 10–15 minutes until the kidneys are tender. Check the seasoning and add more liquid, if necessary, to give the right consistency. Pour into a hot serving dish and serve hot.

MICROWAVE
The sauce can be microwaved but use less liquid.
Not recommended for the kidneys.

SUGGESTED VEGETABLES
Rice, new potatoes or Potato Quiche (page 191). Cauliflower, leeks, courgettes or Brussels sprouts.

BEEF CARBONNADE

Serves 4
Cooking time 2–2¹/2 hours
Oven 180°C, 350°F, Gas Mark 4

This stew comes from the north-eastern region of France and is typical of many from that region. The beer makes a deliciously rich gravy.

450–550 g (1–1¹/4 lb) chuck or bladebone steak
450 g (1 lb) onions
1 clove garlic or ¹/2 teaspoon garlic paste
1 tablespoon brown sugar
1 tablespoon flour
600 ml (1 pint) brown ale
salt and black pepper

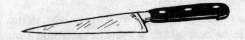

1. Trim the meat of all fat and sinew and cut into 2.5 cm (1 inch) cubes. Peel the onions and garlic. Finely slice the onions and crush the garlic.
2. Dry-fry the meat in a hot frying-pan about one-third at a time until it is browned on all sides (page 245). Remove the meat from the pan and add the onions and sugar. Cook until the sugar caramelizes and browns the onions. You need to have patience and cook them slowly as the browned onions add flavour.
3. Add the garlic and the flour and mix in well. Add the brown ale a little at a time, stirring well so that the flour does not form lumps. Return the meat to the pan and season to taste with salt and black pepper. Transfer the meat to an ovenproof casserole dish, cover and place in a preheated oven at 180°C, 350°F, Gas Mark 4 for 2–2¹/2 hours until the meat is tender.

4. Remove the meat from the pan and place in a hot serving dish. Cover and keep hot. Boil the sauce rapidly to reduce it by one-third. Pour over the meat and serve hot.

MICROWAVE
Can be microwaved on a simmer setting but reduce the liquid.

SUGGESTED VEGETABLES
New or mashed potatoes (with skimmed milk or
low-fat natural yogurt) or Herby Mashed Potatoes (page 200).
Brussels sprouts, cabbage, cauliflower, carrots,
peas or runner beans.

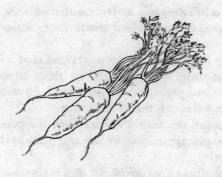

SPICY PINEAPPLE LAMB STEAKS

Serves 4
Cooking time 15–20 minutes

1 clove garlic
1 teaspoon honey
1 teaspoon French mustard
1/2 teaspoon powdered cinnamon
2 teaspoons lemon juice
black pepper
4 lamb steaks, approximately 100–150 g (4–5 oz), cut from the leg
1 x 225 g (8 oz) can pineapple slices in unsweetened juice
salt
1/2 bunch watercress, to garnish

1. Peel and crush the garlic and mix with the honey, French mustard, powdered cinnamon and lemon juice. Season with black pepper.
2. Trim any fat from the lamb steaks and coat with the garlic and honey mixture. Allow to stand for about 20 minutes. Place the steaks under a preheated hot grill for 15–20 minutes, turning them half-way through the cooking time.
3. In the meantime, drain the juice from the pineapple into a pan. Cut the pineapple slices in half and place in the pan. Heat through gently.
4. When the steaks are cooked, arrange them on a hot dish and garnish them around the edge of the dish with the half slices of pineapple. Add the watercress to the dish just before serving. Serve hot.

MICROWAVE
The fruit can be heated in microwave but do not microwave the meat.

SUGGESTED VEGETABLES
Dry Roast Potatoes (page 194) or new potatoes. Cauliflower, cabbage, peas, beans, broccoli or Crispy Courgettes (page 206).

ARMENIAN LAMB CASSEROLE
WITH RICE PILAFF

Serves 4
Cooking time 1–1¼ hours
Oven 180°C, 350°F, Gas Mark 4

This is another dish with a Middle-Eastern flavour. It has delicious blend of spices but use them sparingly the first time you make this dish. You can always vary the flavour to suit yourself. If you prefer, you can substitute 1 teaspoon Garam Masala for the turmeric, cloves, coriander and cinnamon but I think you will prefer your own mixture of spices.

450–550g (1–1¼ lb) lean lamb without bones
2 medium onions
1 clove garlic or ½ teaspoon garlic paste
1 tablespoon flour
1 teaspoon ground cumin seed
½ scant teaspoon allspice
¼ teaspoon turmeric
pinch ground cloves
¼ teaspoon ground coriander
¼ teaspoon ground cinnamon
450 ml (15 fl oz) lamb or beef stock
2 tablespoons tomato purée
salt and black pepper
2 teaspoons white wine vinegar

1. Trim the meat, removing all fat and cut into 2.5 cm (1 inch) dice. Peel the onions and garlic. Slice the onions and crush the garlic.
2. Dry-fry the meat in two to three batches in a hot frying-pan (page 245). Remove the meat from the pan, add the onions and cook for a few minutes, then stir in the flour and spices. Mix well and add the stock a little at a time, stirring well so that the flour does not form lumps. Stir in the tomato purée and season to taste

---

with salt and black pepper. Transfer to an ovenproof dish and cook in a preheated oven at 180°C, 350°F, Gas Mark 4 for 1–1¼ hours or until the meat is tender.

3. In the meantime, make the Rice Pilaff (below).

4. When the meat is cooked remove it from the sauce and place it on a hot serving dish. Cover and keep hot. Check the consistency of the sauce and boil it rapidly (if necessary) to reduce it to a coating consistency. Add the vinegar to the sauce, check the seasoning and pour over the meat.

MICROWAVE
The meat can be microwaved on a simmer setting using a reduced amount of liquid but I find it almost as quick to cook the meat and the rice at the same time in a conventional oven.

SUGGESTED VEGETABLES
French beans, peas, cauliflower, carrots or broccoli.

RICE PILAFF

Serves 4
Cooking time 30–35 minutes
Oven 180°C, 350°F, Gas Mark 4

50 g (2 oz) currants
1 medium onion
1 small red or green pepper
450 ml (15 fl oz) chicken stock
175–225 g (6–8 oz) long-grain rice
2 tablespoons brandy, optional
1 tablespoon chopped parsley

1. Place the currants in a small bowl. Cover them with boiling water and let them soak. Peel and finely chop the onion. Remove the stalk, pith and seeds from the pepper and cut the flesh into small dice.

2. Cook the onion in the chicken stock for 5–7 minutes until it is almost tender. Add the rice and season to taste. Transfer to an ovenproof dish and cover with a lid. Place in a preheated oven at 180°C, 350°F, Gas Mark 4 for 30–35 minutes until the rice is tender. If necessary, add a little more stock during the cooking time but do not stir the rice until it is cooked through. Blanch the pepper in boiling, salted water for 3–4 minutes so that is tender but still has a 'bite', and reserve.

3. When the rice is cooked and the liquid absorbed, drain the currants and stir them into the rice with the pepper and the brandy, if used. Cover and keep hot.

4. Stir the parsley into the rice just before serving. Serve separately with the Armenian Lamb Casserole or, if you wish, make the rice into a border and pour the lamb into the centre. Serve hot.

MICROWAVE
The rice can be microwaved if you prefer.

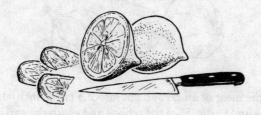

PORK WITH PAPRIKA

Serves 4
Cooking time 1–1¼ hours
Oven 180°C, 350°F, Gas Mark 4

450–550 g (1–1¼ lb) lean pork
2 medium onions
2 cloves garlic or 1 teaspoon garlic paste
100g (4 oz) mushrooms
1 tablespoon flour
50 ml (2 fl oz) dry sherry
300 ml (10 fl oz) chicken stock
1 bay leaf
3 teaspoons paprika
1 tablespoon tomato purée
salt and black pepper
3 tablespoons low-fat fromage frais or low-fat natural yogurt

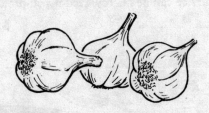

1. Trim the meat of all fat and cut into 2.5 cm (1 inch) dice. Peel the onions and garlic. Slice the onions and crush the garlic. Trim, clean and slice the mushrooms.

2. Dry-fry the meat in a hot frying-pan until it is well coloured on all sides (page 245). Add the flour and mix in well, then pour on the sherry and stock a little at a time, stirring well to prevent lumps of flour forming. Add the bay leaf and stir in the paprika and the tomato purée. Season to taste with salt and black pepper and if necessary transfer to an ovenproof dish. Cook in a pre-heated oven at 180°C, 350°F, Gas Mark 4 for 1–1¼ hours until the meat is tender.

3. Remove the bay leaf from the dish and pour in the fromage frais or yogurt. Heat through gently without boiling. Pour into a hot serving dish and sprinkle a little extra paprika over just before serving.

MICROWAVE
Can be microwaved on a simmer setting but heat conventionally after adding the fromage frais or yogurt.

SUGGESTED VEGETABLES
Rice, egg-free noodles or boiled potatoes. Cauliflower, Oriental Cabbage (page 199), Brussels sprouts or runner beans.

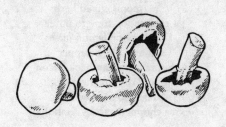

BRAISED STUFFED LIVER

Serves 4
Cooking time 40–45 minutes
Oven 180°C, 350°F, Gas Mark 4

Ask your butcher to cut the liver into long, thin pieces – the wider the better.

4 x 75–100 g (3–4 oz) slices lamb's liver or 8 smaller slices
1 medium onion
1 clove garlic or 1/2 teaspoon garlic paste, optional
2–3 tablespoons fresh breadcrumbs
1 tablespoon chopped parsley
1/2 teaspoon mixed herbs
1 tablespoon tomato purée
1 tablespoon lemon juice
salt and black pepper
4 thin rashers lean back bacon
300 ml (10 fl oz) beef stock
1 teaspoon arrowroot
extra chopped parsley, optional

1. Trim the liver and remove any veins or sinews.
2. Peel the onion and garlic. Grate the onion and crush the garlic. Mix together the onion and garlic with the breadcrumbs, parsley, mixed herbs, tomato purée and the lemon juice. Season well with salt and black pepper.
3. Remove any fat from the bacon and stretch each rasher with the back of a knife so that it will be long enough to wrap around the liver. Lay a piece of liver on each bacon rasher and place an equal amount of stuffing on each. Fold the slice of liver over the top or cover with another piece of liver. Wrap the bacon around and secure each one with cocktail sticks or string.
4. Place the liver parcels in an ovenproof dish and pour the stock over. Cover with a lid and cook in a preheated oven at 180°C, 350°F, Gas Mark 4 for 40–45 minutes until the liver is tender.

5. When the liver is cooked, remove the string or cocktail sticks and place on a hot serving dish. Mix the arrowroot with a little water. Pour the cooking liquor into a small pan and add the arrowroot. Bring to the boil, stirring all the time. Pour a little over the liver and serve the rest separately. If you wish, sprinkle the chopped parsley over the top just before serving. Serve hot.

MICROWAVE
Do not microwave.

SUGGESTED VEGETABLES
New or mashed potatoes (with skimmed milk or
low-fat natural yogurt) or Potato Quiche (page 191).
Carrots, leeks or any green vegetable.

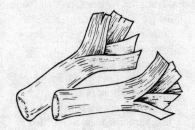

HAM AND PRAWN ROLLS

Serves 4
Cooking time 10–12 minutes

This is an ideal lunch or supper dish and is also good for buffet parties. If it is used on a buffet table it is a good idea to cut the rolls into 2 or 3 pieces to make them easier to handle, and garnish with extra whole prawns around the dish.

100 g (4 oz) long-grain rice
2 tomatoes
1 small green pepper
150 g (6 oz) peeled prawns
2 teaspoons chopped capers, optional
2 tablespoons Tomato Oil-free Dressing (page 237) or
Oil-Free Vinaigrette (page 239)
1/2 tablespoon chopped parsley
1/2 tablespoon chopped chives
salt and black pepper
4 large slices lean ham
4–8 whole prawns
1 lemon, to garnish
a few lettuce leaves, to garnish

1. Cook the rice in boiling, salted water for 10–12 minutes or until just tender. Drain and cool under the cold tap. Drain well.
2. Skin (page 246), and de-seed the tomatoes. Remove the core, pith and seeds from the pepper. Cut the tomatoes and pepper into small dice.
3. Mix together the rice, tomatoes, pepper, peeled prawns and capers if used. Stir in the Tomato Oil-free Dressing or Oil-Free Vinaigrette and the chopped parsley and chives. Season well with salt and black pepper.
4. Place equal portions of the rice mixture on each slice of ham and roll up evenly to enclose the filling.

5. Pull the shells from the tails of the whole prawns. Cut the lemon into wedges. Line a dish with lettuce leaves and place the ham rolls in a row on the lettuce. Garnish with the whole prawns and the lemon wedges. Cover and refrigerate until required.

MICROWAVE
The rice can be microwaved, if preferred.

SUGGESTED VEGETABLES
Extra green or mixed salad, Orange and Onion Salad (page 187) or Chicory and Apple Salad (page 186).

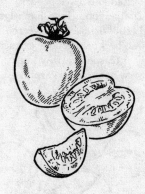

LAMB WITH CRUSTY HERB TOPPING

Serves 4
Cooking time 20–25 minutes
Oven 220°C, 425°F, Gas Mark 7

4 x 100–175 g (4–6 oz) lamb steaks cut from the leg
1–2 cloves garlic or ½–1 teaspoon garlic paste
2–3 tablespoons fresh breadcrumbs
1 tablespoon chopped parsley
salt and black pepper
1–2 tablespoons French mustard
300 ml (10 fl oz) beef or vegetable stock
½–1 teaspoon beef or vegetable extract, optional
1 teaspoon arrowroot
watercress, to garnish

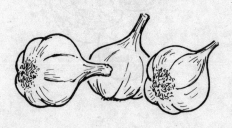

1. Trim any fat from the lamb and place it under a preheated hot grill or cook in a very hot frying-pan or cast-iron grillade for 2–3 minutes to seal each side. Then place in a roasting tin. Peel and crush the garlic, mix with the breadcrumbs and chopped parsley and season well with salt and black pepper.
2. Spread a good layer of French mustard over each lamb steak and cover each one thickly with the breadcrumb mixture. Maintenance Dieters only can dot a little low-fat spread over the top. Cook in a preheated oven at 220°C, 425°F, Gas Mark 7 for

about 20 minutes until the meat is cooked and the topping is nicely browned. If you wish you can place the finished dish under a hot grill to give more colour.

3. Arrange the lamb steaks on a hot serving dish and keep hot. Add the stock to the juices in the pan and stir around well to mix in all the flavouring and any of the topping which remains in the pan. Taste and add a little beef or vegetable extract if you wish. Pour the stock into a small pan, mix the arrowroot with a little water and add to the pan. Bring to the boil stirring all the time. Serve in a sauceboat and garnish the lamb steaks with the watercress just before serving.

MICROWAVE
Do not microwave.

SUGGESTED VEGETABLES
Dry Roast Potatoes (page 194) or Oven Sauté
Potatoes (page 196). Any green vegetable.

BACON AND MUSHROOM ROULADE

Serves 5–6 as a starter, 3–4 as a main course
Cooking time 20–30 minutes plus 15–20 minutes reheating time
Oven 180°C, 350°F, Gas Mark 4

This is another excellent lunch or supper dish. It can also be served as a starter for a special occasion. Vegetarians can substitute 50 g (2 oz) low-fat Cheddar cheese for the bacon.

225 g (8 oz) mushrooms
300 ml (10 fl oz) chicken or vegetable stock
75 g (3 oz) lean back bacon
40 g (1½ oz) cornflour
225 ml (7½ fl oz) skimmed milk
salt and black pepper
2 eggs

1. Line a 28 cm x 18 cm (11 x 7 inch) shallow cake tin or swiss roll tin with lightly oiled greaseproof or silicone paper.
2. Clean and trim the mushrooms and cook them in the stock for 7–8 minutes until they are tender. Remove from the stock with a draining spoon and drain well. Reserve the stock. Chop the mushrooms coarsely.
3. Remove any fat from the bacon and cut into strips or dice. Cook in the stock for 3–4 minutes, then remove (reserving the stock). Chop coarsely and mix with half the mushrooms.
4. Boil the stock until it reduces to 65 ml (2½ fl oz). Mix the cornflour with a little of the milk. Add the rest of the milk to the stock and bring to the boil. Pour on to the cornflour, mix well and return to the pan. Bring to the boil and cook for 2–3 minutes, stirring all the time. Season to taste with salt and pepper.
5. Place half the sauce in a large bowl and stir in the bacon and mushroom mixture. Stir the remainder of the mushrooms into the rest of the sauce and reserve.

6. Separate the eggs and beat the egg yolks into the bacon and mushroom mixture. Whisk the egg whites until they stand in stiff peaks. Fold one tablespoon into the eggs, bacon and mushroom mixture really well to loosen the texture then fold in the remainder very lightly in two to three batches.

7. Pour the mixture into the prepared tin. Spread it lightly so that it is an even thickness. Place in a preheated oven at 180°C, 350°F , Gas Mark 4 for 20–30 minutes until it springs back like a sponge and shrinks away from the sides of the tin.

8. Turn out on to a clean tea towel and carefully lift off the tin. Leave to cool for about five minutes then ease off the paper, using a palette knife if necessary. Trim a thin slice from each of the short ends.

9. Have one of the long edges of the roulade base towards you and spread the reserved mushroom mixture over half the base nearest to you. Lift the tea towel and pull it away from you so that the base rolls up like a swiss roll. Slip an ovenproof plate under the roulade and roll it on to the plate with the open seam underneath.

10. Maintenance Dieters and vegetarians can sprinkle a little grated low-fat cheese down the length of the roulade.

11. To serve, reheat in a preheated oven at 180°C, 350°F, Gas Mark 4 for 12–15 minutes. Serve hot.

MICROWAVE
Make conventionally but can be reheated in a microwave.

SUGGESTED VEGETABLES
Serve with a salad.

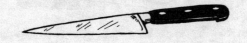

GRILLED MEATS WITH SPECIAL SAVOURY SAUCES

Grilling is an excellent way to cook meats on the Hip and Thigh Diet. To make them more interesting serve with no-fat sauces, as listed below.

Grilling times: (remember to turn all meats half-way through the cooking times and the grill must be very hot before starting to cook)
Lamb's liver: 5–8 minutes, depending on thickness
Lamb chops or steaks 2–2.5 cm (¾–1 inch) thick: 10–15 minutes
Pork chops 2-2.5 cm (¾–1 inch thick): 15–20 minutes
Bacon rashers (thin): 3–5 minutes
Gammon rasher of steaks 1 cm (½ inch) thick: 7–10 minutes
Ham steaks 1 cm (½ inch) thick: 7–10 minutes
Steak 2–2.5 cm (¾–1 inch) thick: rare 5 minutes;
   medium rare 7–8 minutes; well done 12 minutes
Minute steak: 0.5–1 cm (¼–½ inch) thick: 3–4 minutes

Serve liver or lamb with Spicy Raisin Sauce (page 241)
Serve pork, bacon or ham with Cumberland Sauce (page 242)
Serve steak with Fromage Frais and Horseradish Sauce (page 240)

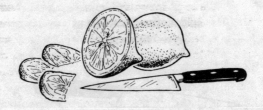

BOILED BEEF WITH HORSERADISH SAUCE

Cold meat cooked in this way is delicious with salads.

Serves 5–6
Cooking time 45 minutes per 450 g (1 lb) plus 45 minutes (minimum cooking time 2¹/₂–3 hours)
Oven 160°C, 325°F, Gas Mark 3

1.5 kg (3–3¹/₂ lb) joint salt silverside of beef
5–6 small onions or 10–12 pickling onions
5–6 carrots
2–3 parsnips, optional
3–4 leeks
3–4 sticks celery, optional
1–2 bay leaves
1 quantity Fromage Frais and Horseradish Sauce (page 240)
¹/₂ quantity Pease Pudding, see below, optional

1. Remove the outer layer of fat from around the joint. Re-tie to a neat shape and weigh to calculate the cooking time.
2. Peel the onions, carrots and parsnips. Cut the carrots into four lengthways and the parsnips into large pieces. Trim and wash the leeks and celery sticks and cut each into two to three pieces.
3. Place the meat in a large heatproof casserole or pan with the prepared vegetables. Add the bay leaves and cover with water. Bring slowly to the boil then transfer to a preheated oven at 160°C, 325°F, Gas Mark 3 and cook, allowing 45 minutes per 450 g (1 lb) plus an extra 45 minutes. Or if you wish you can simmer the meat gently on top of the stove for the same time.
4. When the meat is cooked, remove it from the casserole or pan and discard the bay leaves. Remove the string and slice the meat. Arrange it on a hot serving dish with the vegetables around the sides. If you prefer, you can serve some of the vegetables sepa-

---

rately. Pour some of the cooking liquor into a sauceboat (if you wish you can thicken it with arrowroot) and serve separately with the meat and Fromage Frais and Horseradish Sauce, and the Pease Pudding if you wish.

MICROWAVE
Microwaving is not recommended.

SUGGESTED VEGETABLES
No other vegetables other than potatoes are necessary.

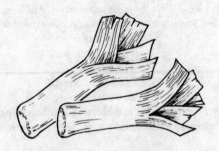

PEASE PUDDING

1 quantity Split Pea Purée (page 205) – use yellow split peas
1 egg
salt and black pepper

Make the Split Pea Purée, beat in the egg and season to taste with salt and black pepper. Place in a lightly oiled pudding basin and stand it in a pan. Pour boiling water into the pan until it comes half-way up the basin and steam for 30–45 minutes. Alternatively, place the purée in a dish and bake in a preheated oven at 180°C, 350°F, Gas Mark 4 for about 30 minutes. Leftover Pease Pudding can be reheated and served with cold meat the next day, or can be made into a soup with any remaining vegetables and the cooking liquor.

HONEYED PORK
WITH TAGLIATELLE

Tricolour tagliatelle looks very attractive with this dish but do take care that any pasta you use is not made with eggs. If you can not find any tomato passata use canned tomatoes. They are nicer if you purée them and then sieve them to remove the seeds.

Serves 4
Cooking time 20–25 minutes

2 medium onions
100 g (4 oz) mushrooms
450 ml (15 fl oz) tomato passata
1 chicken stockcube
salt and black pepper
450 g (1 lb) pork fillet or thin pork escalopes
2 teaspoons clear honey
1 tablespoon soy sauce
225–275 g (8–10 oz) tagliatelle

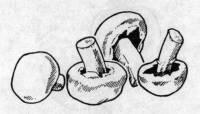

1. Peel and finely chop the onions. Clean, trim and slice the mushrooms. Pour the tomato passata into a pan and add the stockcube and onions. Heat gently and stir until the stockcube has dissolved, then simmer slowly until the onions are almost tender. Add the mushrooms and continue cooking for another 4–5 minutes until the mushrooms and onions are cooked. Taste and, if necessary, season with salt and pepper.

2. In the meantime, cut the pork fillet into thin slices then cut the sliced fillet or the escalopes into thin strips. Dry-fry (page 245) quickly in a hot frying-pan. A wok is ideal if you have one. When the pork is nicely coloured, stir in the honey and the soy sauce. Mix well to ensure that the pork strips are well coated. Pour the tomato mixture on to the pork, mix well and gently cook for a further 3–4 minutes or until the pork is tender.

3. Cook the tagliatelle in boiling, salted water. Consult the packet for the cooking time. Drain well and pile on to a hot dish or individual dishes. Make a well in the centre of the tagliatelle and pour in the pork. Serve hot.

MICROWAVE

Do not microwave the meat. The tagliatelle can be microwaved if you prefer.

SUGGESTED VEGETABLES

Broccoli, peas, beans, cauliflower or courgettes.

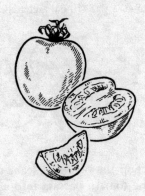

GUINNESS HOT-POT

Serves 4–5
Cooking time 3–3½ hours
Oven 160°C, 325°F, Gas Mark 3

450–600 g (1–1¼ lb) lean chuck or bladebone steak
2 large onions
3 large carrots
750 g (1½ lb) small old potatoes
450 g (1 lb) leeks
2–3 celery sticks
1 teaspoon sugar
40 g (1½ oz) flour
salt and black pepper
1 x 400 ml (14 fl oz) can Guinness
450 ml (15 fl oz) beef stock
1 tablespoon tomato purée

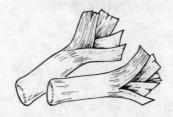

1. Trim the meat and remove any sinew and fat. Cut into 2.5 cm (1 inch) dice. Peel the onion, carrots and potatoes. Slice them into moderately thin slices. Trim and wash the leeks and celery. Cut them into 1 cm (½ inch) pieces.

2. Dry-fry the onions and carrots with the sugar. Cook until they are golden brown (page 245). Remove the vegetables from the pan and dry-fry the meat over a good heat. Stir the flour into the meat.

3. Layer the carrots and onions, leeks, celery, meat and potatoes in a 2.25 litre (4 pint) casserole dish. Season each layer with salt and black pepper. End with a layer of potatoes.

4. Mix the Guinness and stock together with the tomato purée. Bring to the boil, check the seasoning and pour into the casserole. Cover and cook in a preheated oven at 160°C, 325°F, Gas Mark 3 for 3–3½ hours until the vegetables and meat are tender. Press the top layer of potatoes into the gravy occasionally while they are cooking and add a little more stock if necessary to prevent them drying out. Remove the lid and allow the potatoes to crisp and brown for the last 15 minutes of cooking. Serve in the cooking pot.

MICROWAVE
Can be microwaved on a simmer setting but use less liquid. Finish in a conventional oven or under a hot grill to crisp and brown the potatoes.

SUGGESTED VEGETABLES
Carrot and Parsnip Purée (page 204), cabbage, Brussels sprouts or spring greens.

Vegetarian

More people are becoming interested in vegetarian recipes, both those who wish to cut out meat and its products completely and others to give a change from their normal diet. Whoever uses these recipes, I hope they will enjoy them but a word of warning to any dieter using this section occasionally. As Rosemary explains in her introduction (page 9), because vegetarian meals contain little natural fat, some licence in given in these recipes to ensure that they provide a well-balanced diet, and so some fat is included. Although Rosemary explains that an occasional break will do little harm to non-vegetarian dieters, I would suggest that they avoid the Cottage and Cheddar Cheese Bake (page 173) and, if they want to use any of these recipes on a regular basis, they should omit the oil and cook by the dry-fry methods (page 245) I use in all the other sections.

I have tried to include a good number of recipes to appeal to vegans. Care has been taken to ensure a proper balance of proteins in all the recipes intended as main meals. I hope that all vegetarians will find this section useful to their diet.

I also hope that they will not confine their use of this book to this chapter alone. They will find that many other recipes in this book will be suitable: even in the meat chapter there are recipes such as the Bacon and Mushroom Roulade (page 142) which can be adapted. The Soups and Starters chapter and the Salads and Vegetables chapter will provide many more recipes which can be used either just as they are or with slight adjustments to suit your needs and provide greater variety both for family meals and for entertaining.

Vegetarian

Ⓥ suitable for vegetarians
Ⓑ budget-conscious recipe
Ⓠ quick to prepare and cook

VEGETABLE TERRINE

Serves 6 as a starter, 4 as a main course
Cooking time 40–45 minutes
Oven 180°C, 350°F, Gas Mark 4

Sorrel is a green herb which looks like small spinach leaves. It grows wild, is easy to grow in the garden and is often available in supermarkets and ethnic shops. It has a slightly bitter taste which contrasts well with the other ingredients in this terrine. If you are unable to obtain sorrel, use spinach and add a little lemon juice.

450 g (1 lb) small courgettes
150 g (5 oz) fresh sorrel or spinach
2 eggs
50 g (2 oz) grated Gruyère cheese
2 teaspoons
lemon juice (or to taste) if spinach is used
salt and black pepper
1 quantity Three Vegetable Fondue (page 243), to serve

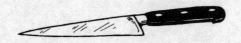

1. Lightly oil the inside of a 450 g (1 lb) terrine or loaf tin. Line the base with greaseproof paper.
2. Trim the courgettes and cook whole in boiling, salted water for 7–8 minutes. Drain well and place under cold running water until they are completely cold. Drain well again. Quarter each courgette lengthways and slice thickly.
3. Remove any coarse stalks from the sorrel or spinach. Blanch the sorrel in boiling, salted water for 1–2 minutes and the spinach for 3–4 minutes. Sorrel has very tender leaves so needs very little cooking. Drain the sorrel or spinach very well, then return to

the pan and stir over a gentle heat for a minute or two to dry out the moisture. Remove from the heat. Beat the eggs well and mix with the sorrel or spinach, courgettes and the cheese. Season to taste and add lemon juice if spinach was used. Pour into the prepared terrine or tin and cook in a preheated oven at 180°C, 350°F, Gas Mark 4 for 40 minutes or until the terrine is firm and shrinking slightly from the sides of the dish. Remove from the oven, cool and then refrigerate. Turn out and slice. Serve on individual plates with a little Three Vegetable Fondue sauce on each side of the sliced terrine.

FREEZING
This terrine can be frozen very satisfactorily but the sauce should be freshly made.

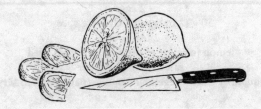

HUMMUS

Serves 4

This makes an excellent starter as well as a lunch dish.

1 x 400 g (14 oz) can chick peas
3 cloves garlic or 1½ teaspoons garlic paste
3 lemons or 100–150 ml (3–5 fl oz) lemon juice
5 tablespoons tahini paste
5 tablespoons low-fat natural yogurt
pinch cayenne
salt

1. Drain the chick peas and reserve the liquid. Peel and crush the garlic. Place the chick peas and garlic in a food processor or liquidizer with 4 tablespoons of the reserved liquid. Process until smooth.

2. Add 100 ml (3½ fl oz) lemon juice, the tahini paste and the yogurt. Process again until well mixed. Season to taste with a pinch of cayenne, salt and a little more lemon juice, and/or some reserved liquid if desired, to give the right consistency.

3. Turn out into a bowl and serve with a salad or crudités and small pitta bread.

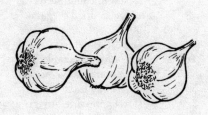

RED BEAN AND BURGUNDY CASSEROLE

Serves 4
Cooking time 40–50 minutes plus soaking time

If using dried red kidney beans they must be soaked in cold water for at least 5 hours or overnight. Then drain and rinse them well. Place in a pan and cover with water. Bring to the boil and BOIL RAPIDLY FOR 15 MINUTES. This is essential. Lower the heat and simmer gently for 1¼–2 hours until the beans are tender. It is also essential that the beans are completely cooked before they are eaten. Do not add salt until the beans are cooked, otherwise they will toughen.

100 g (4 oz) dried red kidney beans or
1 x 225 g (8 oz) can red beans
75 g (3 oz) dried brown or green lentils (page 111)
1 medium onion
1 clove garlic or ½ teaspoon garlic paste
2 medium potatoes
100 g (4 oz) carrot
2 leeks
100 g (4 oz) mushrooms
2 tablespoons olive oil
1 teaspoon cumin seeds
½ teaspoon dried oregano
1 x 200 g (7 oz) can tomatoes
300 ml (10 fl oz) red wine
65 ml (2½ fl oz) vegetable stock
1 tablespoon tomato purée
1 bay leaf
¼–½ teaspoon dried thyme
salt and black pepper
6–8 small florets cauliflower
chopped parsley, to garnish

1. If dried beans are used, soak and cook them as above. If canned beans are used, drain and rinse them well.

2. Wash the lentils, drain, place in a pan of cold water, bring to the boil and simmer for 15–20 minutes. Drain and reserve the lentils and the cooking liquid.

3. Peel the onion, garlic, potatoes and carrots. Trim and wash the leeks. Chop the onions and crush the garlic. Cut the potatoes into large dice and place in cold water until required. Thickly slice the carrots and leeks. Clean and trim the mushrooms.

4. Heat the oil in a large heavy pan and cook the onion and garlic until they are soft. Add the cumin and oregano and cook for a further 2 minutes. Add the lentils to the pan with the dried cooked beans (if used), tomatoes, red wine, stock, tomato purée, bay leaf and thyme. Cover and simmer for 10–12 minutes. Add the potatoes and carrots and season lightly. Simmer for a further 10 minutes, then add the cauliflower, leeks, mushrooms and canned red beans (if used). Continue cooking for a further 8–10 minutes. If necessary add a little more of the cooking liquid from the lentils to the pan to keep the vegetables moist.

5. When all the vegetables are tender, check the seasoning, remove the bay leaf and pile into a hot serving dish. Sprinkle chopped parsley over just before serving. Serve hot.

MICROWAVE
Cook dried beans conventionally. The rest of the dish can be microwaved.

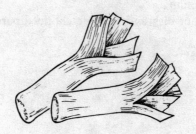

SAVOURY BROWN RICE

Serves 4
Cooking time 35–40 minutes

This makes a tasty dish to accompany many main courses.

1 large onion
100–175 g (4–6 oz) green pepper
100–175 g (4–6 oz) red pepper
1 stick celery
1 x 400 (14 oz) can chopped tomatoes
300 ml (10 fl oz) vegetable stock
225 g (8 oz) brown rice
salt and black pepper
chopped parsley, to garnish

1. Peel and finely chop the onion. Remove the stalk, pith and seeds from the peppers. (You need about 100 g (4 oz) of each after they have been trimmed.) Wash and trim the celery. Cut the peppers and the celery into 1 cm (1/2 inch) dice.
2. Place the vegetables in a pan with the tomatoes, stock and the rice. Season with 1/2 teaspoon salt and black pepper. Bring to the boil and simmer gently for 30–35 minutes until the rice is tender. Stir occasionally to prevent the rice sticking to the pan. Add a little water or more stock if necessary to keep the rice moist but all the liquid should evaporate by the time the rice is cooked. Check the seasoning.
3. Pile into a hot dish and sprinkle chopped parsley over just before serving.

SPINACH ROULADE

Serves 6–8 as a starter, 4–5 as a main course
Cooking time 35–45 minutes
Oven 180°C, 350°F, Gas Mark 4

This can be served as a spectacular starter or main dish.

750 g (1½ lb) fresh spinach or
350g (12 oz) frozen leaf spinach (page 63)
50 g (2 oz) cornflour
450ml (15 fl oz) skimmed milk
salt and black pepper
3 eggs
good pinch nutmeg
75 g (3 oz) grated low-fat Cheddar cheese

1. Line a 30 x 20 cm (12 x 8 in) non-stick swiss roll tin with lightly oiled greaseproof or silicone paper.
2. Wash the fresh spinach well and remove any coarse stalks. Cook in boiling water for 6–7 minutes until tender. Cook frozen spinach for 2–3 minutes. Drain well, using a potato masher to squeeze out as much water as possible. Chop very finely.
2. Mix the cornflour with a little milk. Bring the rest of the milk to the boil. Pour a little on to the cornflour, stir well and return to the pan, and bring to the boil, stirring all the time. Boil for 2–3 minutes. Season well with salt and pepper and a good pinch of nutmeg.
3. Measure the sauce and pour half into a large bowl and stir in the spinach. Beat most of the cheese into the remainder of the sauce and reserve for later.
4. Separate the eggs and beat the yolks into the sauce in the bowl with the spinach. Whisk the egg whites until they stand in stiff peaks and fold one tablespoon into the spinach mixture very well to loosen it, then fold in the remainder lightly in two or three batches.

5. Pour the mixture into the prepared tin, tipping it from side to side to fill the tin evenly. Avoid spreading it with a spatula if possible, as this will break down the air bubbles. Cook in a preheated oven at 180°C, 350°F, Gas Mark 4 for 20–25 minutes until the mixture is set and springy like a sponge and is pulling away from the sides of the tin.

6. Turn the roulade on to a clean tea towel and carefully remove the tin. Leave for about 5 minutes, then carefully peel off the paper, using a palette knife if necessary.

7. Trim a thin slice off each of the narrow ends and have one of the long edges of the roulade towards you. Beat the reserved cheese sauce well and spread over the two-thirds of the roulade nearest to you. Lift the edge of the tea towel which is in front of you and pull it away from you so that the roulade rolls up like a swiss roll. Try to roll it as tightly as possible so that there is no gap in the middle. Slip an ovenproof plate under the roulade so that the seam is underneath. Sprinkle the remainder of the cheese over the top.

8. When you wish to eat the roulade, place it in a preheated oven at 180°C, 350°F, Gas Mark 4 for 12–15 minutes until it is heated through and the cheese on top has melted. Serve hot.

MICROWAVE
Make the roulade in the conventional way but it can be
reheated in the microwave.

FREEZING
It can be frozen after step 7.

SPICED LENTILS AND CHICK PEAS

Serves 4
Cooking time 20–25 minutes

225 g (8 oz) onions
225 g (8 oz) carrots
2 cloves garlic or 1 teaspoon garlic paste
2 sticks celery
1 small red pepper
225 g (8 oz) orange lentils
450 ml (15 fl oz) vegetable stock
2–3 teaspoons curry powder (to taste)
pinch ground cloves
1/2 teaspoon ground coriander
1/2 teaspoon cinnamon powder
1 tablespoon tomato purée
1 x 400 g (14 oz) can chick peas
salt and black pepper
300 ml (10 fl oz) low-fat natural yogurt

1. Peel the onions, carrots and garlic. Trim and wash the celery. Remove the stalk, pith and seeds from the pepper. Dice the onions, carrots, celery and pepper. Crush the garlic.
2. Wash the lentils and place in a pan with the vegetables and garlic. Pour on the stock and stir in the curry powder, cloves, coriander, cinnamon and the tomato purée. Bring to the boil, cover and simmer gently for 20–25 minutes until the lentils are tender. Drain and rinse the chick peas and stir into the pan. Cook for a further 8–10 minutes or until all the liquid has evaporated. Season to taste with salt and black pepper. Pile into a hot serving dish and serve with the yogurt.

MICROWAVE
This dish can be microwaved but I prefer it cooked conventionally.

FREEZING
This dish can be frozen without the yogurt.

VEGETABLE COUSCOUS

Serves 4
Cooking time approximately 1 hour

If you are using easy-cook couscous, consult the packet for cooking directions. Harissa is a very hot pepper paste and is available from some supermarkets and ethnic stores. You can, if you wish, add both dried apricots and raisins to the couscous. Some traditional recipes include a high proportion of dried fruit.

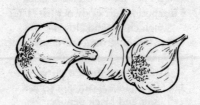

225 g (8 oz) couscous
1 small aubergine
salt
2 medium onions
3 cloves garlic or 1¹/₂ teaspoons garlic paste
1 large firm potato
2 medium carrots
2–3 small courgettes
1 medium green pepper
1–2 chilli peppers
2 tablespoons olive oil
1 x 400 g (14 oz) can chopped tomatoes
black pepper
225 g (8 oz) cooked or canned chick peas
50 g (2 oz) ready-to-cook dried apricots and/or raisins
³/₄ teaspoon ground coriander
³/₄ teaspoon ground cumin
1 teaspoon turmeric
2 hard-boiled eggs, optional
hot pepper sauce or harissa

1. Place the couscous in a large bowl and pour in 300 ml (10 fl oz) cold water, mixing it in gently and lifting the grains with your fingers so that they are all moistened. Drain and leave for 10 minutes and as the grains swell rake them with your fingers from time to time to prevent lumps forming.

2. Place the couscous in a steamer or colander lined with a clean tea towel or muslin. Fold the tea towel over the top, cover with a tight lid and place over a pan of gently boiling water. Steam for 30 minutes.

3. In the meantime, dice the aubergine and sprinkle with 1 teaspoon salt. Place on a wire rack over a bowl or plate and leave for 30 minutes. Rinse in cold water and drain well.

4. Peel the onions, garlic, potato and carrots. Trim the courgettes and remove the stalk, pith and seeds from the pepper. Slice the onions, cut the potato and carrots into large dice and the courgettes into 2.5 cm (1 inch) slices. Cut the pepper into thick strips. Cut the chillies in half lengthways and remove the seeds. If you like a very hot couscous leave the seeds in but, whatever you do, remember to wash your hands after touching the chillies. The juice from them will be very painful if you touch your eyes after handling them.

5. When the couscous has been cooking for 30 minutes, turn it out into a large bowl. Stir the grains gently with a fork or your fingers to break up any lumps and work in the olive oil. Return it to the muslin-lined steamer.

6. Pour away the water from the pan and add the onions, garlic, potato, carrots, courgettes, green pepper, chillies and the tomatoes to the pan with 300 ml (10 fl oz) water, season to taste with salt. Season lightly because the aubergines may add more salt. Replace the steamer over the pan. Continue steaming for 20 minutes, with the vegetables cooking underneath, then add the aubergine, chick peas, apricots (which have been cut into 2–3 pieces) and/or raisins and the spices. Add more water if necessary. Stir the couscous grains again to break up any lumps and continue steaming for a further 10 minutes or until the vegetables are tender.

7. Pile the couscous into a large dish and make a well in the centre. Spoon the vegetables into the centre. Dilute the cooking liquor if necessary to a thin pouring consistency. Pour some into a bowl or sauceboat. Dilute the hot pepper sauce or harissa with a little more liquid. Pour into another bowl or sauceboat. Just before serving, garnish the couscous with slices or wedges of hard-boiled egg (if used). Serve the cooking liquor and hot pepper sauce or harissa separately.

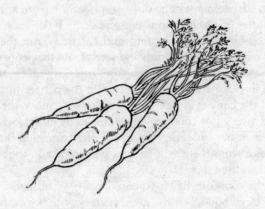

TOMATO AND VEGETABLE RING

Serves 6–8 as a starter, 4–6 as a main course

I used a gelatine substitute based on carrageen for this recipe. The packet stated 1 teaspoon to 600 ml (1 pt) for normal use and 2 teaspoons for acidic liquids. I used 2 teaspoons as I felt the tomato juice and other liquids would be acidic and found it satisfactory but suggest you read the instructions on the packet you use.

2 teaspoons gelatine substitute (see above)
600 ml (1 pint) tomato juice
1 tablespoon lemon juice
1 teaspoon sugar
1 tablespoon Worcestershire Sauce, optional
salt and white pepper
50 g (2 oz) french beans
225–350 g (8–12 oz) small new potatoes
50 g (2 oz) peas
75 g (3 oz) sweetcorn (canned or frozen)
2–3 hard-boiled eggs
1 x 350 g (12 oz) can asparagus spears, optional
2–3 tablespoons Low-fat Salad Cream (page 238)
2–3 tomatoes
a few lettuce leaves, to serve
chopped chives, to garnish

1. Dissolve the gelatine substitute in a little hot water and stir into the tomato juice with the lemon juice, sugar and Worcestershire Sauce (if used). Season with salt and white pepper. Pour a little into a 20 cm (8 inch) ring mould or a 1 litre (2 pint) mould and leave to set.

2. Trim the french beans and cut into 2.5 cm (1 inch) pieces. Scrape the potatoes and cut into 1 cm (1/2 inch) dice. Cook the beans, potatoes, peas and sweetcorn separately in boiling, salted water. Drain all the vegetables well when they are cooked, then place under cold running water until completely cold. Drain well again (page 246).

3. Remove the shells from the hard-boiled eggs. Slice one and arrange decoratively in the base of the ring mould with peas and some of the tips of asparagus between each slice. Pour over a little more jelly and leave to set.

4. Chop the other hard-boiled egg and cut the remainder of the asparagus into short lengths. Mix together all the vegetables except for the potatoes. When the remainder of the jelly is on the point of setting, add the mixed vegetables and egg and pour into the mould. Leave until set.

5. Mix the potato with sufficient Low-fat Salad Cream to coat and reserve. Quarter or slice the tomatoes.

6. Turn the mould out on to a chilled plate. Moisten the plate slightly and you will then be able to position the jelly in the centre of the dish. Fill the centre with the potato salad. Arrange the lettuce leaves and tomato around the edge of the plate and sprinkle chopped chives over the potato. Refrigerate until required.

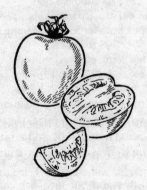

MIDDLE EASTERN PILAFF

Serves 4
Cooking time 35–40 minutes

1 medium aubergine
salt
1 medium onion
2 cloves garlic or 1 teaspoon garlic paste
2 carrots
2 courgettes
1 tablespoon oil
½ teaspoon ground ginger
½ teaspoon ground cardamom
100 g (4 oz) brown rice
600 ml (1 pt) vegetable stock
100 g (4 oz) white easy-cook rice
50 g (2 oz) sultanas
175–225 g (6–8 oz) canned or cooked chick peas
black pepper
1–2 tablespoons Parmesan cheese

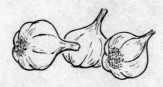

1. Cut the aubergine into 2.5 cm (1 inch) dice. Place on a wire rack over a bowl or plate and sprinkle 1 teaspoon salt over. Leave for 30 minutes then rinse and drain well.

2. Peel the onion, garlic and carrots. Trim the courgettes. Chop the onions, and crush the garlic. Cut the carrots into quarters lengthways and cut the carrots and courgettes into 5 mm (¼ inch) slices.

3. Heat the oil in a heavy pan and add the onion and garlic. Cook gently until soft then add the carrots and courgettes and cook until lightly coloured.

4. Stir in the ground ginger and cardamom and mix well. Then add the brown rice and the stock. Season lightly with salt and bring to the boil. Simmer gently for 20–25 minutes then add the white rice, aubergine, sultanas and the chick peas. Cook for another 12–15 minutes until the rice is tender and all the liquid has been absorbed. If necessary, add a little more stock or water to the rice while it is cooking but make certain it has all been absorbed by the end of the cooking time.

5. Taste and season with pepper and more salt if necessary. Stir in the Parmesan cheese and serve hot.

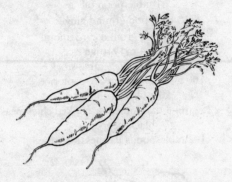

GNOCCHI VERDI WITH FRESH TOMATO SAUCE

Serves 4
Cooking time 15–20 minutes

1 kg (2 lb) fresh spinach or
450 g (1 lb) frozen leaf spinach (page 63)
2 onions
2 cloves garlic or 1 teaspoon garlic paste
2 teaspoons olive oil
2 egg yolks
2 tablespoons flour
4 tablespoons Parmesan cheese
100 g (4 oz) low-fat ricotta or low-fat cottage cheese
2 tablespoons skimmed milk (only required if cottage cheese is used)
pinch nutmeg
salt and black pepper
1 quantity Fresh Tomato Sauce (page 236)
chopped fresh basil

1. Wash the fresh spinach well and remove any coarse stalks. Cook in boiling, salted water. Fresh spinach will take 6–7 minutes, frozen spinach 3–4 minutes. Drain well and use a potato masher to press out as much water as possible.
2. Peel the onions and garlic. Finely chop the onions and crush the garlic. Heat the oil in a pan and cook the onions and garlic until they are soft but without colour. Stir in the spinach and stir it around in the pan until it is completely dry. Remove from the heat and cool.
3. Beat the egg yolks, flour and Parmesan cheese together. Then beat in the ricotta cheese. If cottage cheese is used, purée it in a food processor with the milk. Mix into the spinach with a pinch of nutmeg, and season well with salt and black pepper.
4. Shape into balls about the size of walnuts then flatten them slightly. Cover with food wrap and refrigerate for at least 2 hours

before use. (They can be deep frozen very satisfactorily at this stage. Defrost in the refrigerator or at room temperature then chill in the refrigerator. They are easier to cook if well chilled.)

5. To cook: drop the gnocchi into a large pan of boiling, salted water and simmer for 7–10 minutes. When they are cooked, they rise to the surface. Remove with a draining spoon, cover and keep hot. It is advisable to cook them in batches according to the size of the pan. If you overload the pan, the gnocchi will stick together.

6. In the meantime, make the Fresh Tomato Sauce (page 236). Add some chopped basil and toss the gnocchi in the sauce. Serve hot.

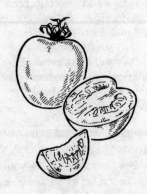

SPAGHETTI AND TOFU BOLOGNAISE

Serves 4
Cooking time 15–20 minutes

1 x 275 g (10 oz) packet tofu
1 medium onion
2 cloves garlic or 1 teaspoon garlic paste
2 sticks celery
1/2 small green pepper
1/2 small red pepper
100 g (4 oz) mushrooms
1 tablespoon oil
1 x 400 g (14 oz) can chopped tomatoes
2 teaspoons tomato purée
150 ml (5 fl oz) vegetable stock
salt and black pepper
275–350 g (10–12 oz) wholewheat spaghetti
2 tablespoons Parmesan cheese

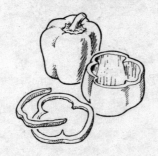

1. Cut the tofu into 1 cm (1/2 inch) dice and leave to drain on kitchen paper.
2. Peel the onion and garlic. Chop the onion and crush the garlic. Trim and wash the celery. Remove the stalks, pith and seeds from the peppers. Cut the celery and peppers into small dice. Trim, clean and slice the mushrooms.

3. Heat the oil in a heavy pan and cook the tofu until it is lightly coloured. Remove from the pan and add the onion, garlic, celery and peppers. Cook gently for a few minutes until they soften but are without colour then stir in the tomatoes, tomato purée, and stock. Season to taste with salt and pepper and add the tofu. Bring to the boil and simmer gently for 10 minutes.

4. Add the mushrooms and cook for a further 10 minutes, cooking rapidly enough to reduce the sauce to a coating consistency.

5. In the meantime, cook the spaghetti in boiling, salted water until just tender. Drain well and place in a large hot serving dish or individual plates. Pour the sauce into the middle of the spaghetti and serve with the Parmesan cheese.

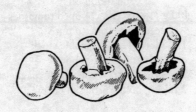

COTTAGE AND CHEDDAR CHEESE BAKE

Serves 4
Cooking time 30–35 minutes
Oven 220°C, 425°F, Gas Mark 7

Even for vegetarians, this recipe is a little high on fat content but it is so delicious it is worth saving for a special occasion. Non-vegetarians should avoid the dish.

100 g (4 oz) mushrooms
150 ml (5 fl oz) vegetable stock
2–3 large tomatoes
350 g (12 oz) low-fat cottage cheese
75–100 g (3–4 oz) grated low-fat Cheddar cheese
3 eggs
salt and black pepper
fresh or dried basil or dried oregano

1. Lightly oil a 600-900 ml (1–1½ pt) pie or soufflé dish.
2. Trim and clean the mushrooms. Cook them in the stock for 5–6 minutes until tender. Drain well. Skin (page 246) and slice the tomatoes.
3. Mix the cottage cheese and Cheddar cheese together in a large bowl. Separate 2 of the eggs and stir the yolks and the remaining egg into the cheese. Mix well and season with salt and black pepper.
4. Whisk the egg whites until they stand in stiff peaks and fold into the mixture. Pour into the prepared dish and cover with the mushrooms and the sliced tomatoes. Season the tomatoes lightly and sprinkle the oregano or basil over.
5. Place in a preheated oven at 220°C, 425°F, Gas Mark 7 for 30–35 minutes until well risen and golden brown.
6. Serve hot with crusty bread and a salad.

STUFFED AUBERGINES

Serves 8 as a starter, 4 as a main dish
Cooking time 35–40 minutes
Oven 180°C, 350°F, Gas Mark 4

This is a traditional Middle Eastern dish with the raisins, sultanas and the spices. However, if you prefer you can use mushrooms instead of the dried fruit. If you wish to serve this with a tomato sauce, either recipe on pages 235 and 236 would be suitable.

4 medium aubergines
salt
50 g (2 oz) raisins or sultanas, or 100 g (4 oz) button mushrooms
2 medium onions
2 large tomatoes
1 tablespoons oil
175 g (6 oz) cooked rice
1 tablespoon chopped mint, parsley or coriander
1/4 teaspoon allspice
1/4 teaspoon cinnamon
black pepper
50–75 g (2–3 oz) grated low-fat Cheddar cheese
1 quantity Tomato Sauce (pages 235 and 236), optional

1. Cut the aubergines in half. With a small, pointed knife make a criss-cross of cuts across the flesh without cutting through the skin. Sprinkle lightly with salt. Place cut side down on a wire rack over a plate or tray and leave for 30 minutes, then rinse well and blanch in a large pan of boiling salted water for 8–10 minutes until the flesh is nearly cooked.
2. Place the raisins or sultanas, if used, in a small bowl, cover with boiling water and leave until required. Peel and finely chop the onions. Skin (page 246), de-seed and chop the tomatoes. Trim, clean and chop the mushrooms, if used.
3. Scoop the centres out of the aubergines. Reserve the skins and

chop the flesh. Drain the raisins or sultanas. Heat the oil in a pan and cook the onions until they are soft and golden brown. Add the mushrooms, if used, cook for 3–4 minutes and then add the tomatoes and the aubergine flesh and cook for another 2–3 minutes. Stir in the cooked rice, chopped herbs, allspice, cinnamon and the raisins or sultanas, if used. Season to taste with salt and black pepper.

4. Pile the mixture into the aubergine skins. Place in an oven-proof dish and sprinkle the grated cheese over the top. Cook in a preheated oven at 180°C, 350°F, Gas Mark 4 for 30 minutes until the aubergines are tender and golden brown. Transfer to a hot serving dish or individual dishes. Serve with Tomato Sauce if you wish.

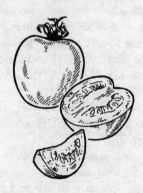

VEGETABLE AND TOFU SALAD

Serves 4–6

2 tablespoons sesame oil
3 tablespoons soy sauce
3 tablespoons white wine vinegar or cider vinegar
2 teaspoons clear honey
1 clove garlic or 1/2 teaspoon garlic paste
2 x 275 g (10 oz) packets tofu
2 sticks celery
50 g (2 oz) white button mushrooms
2–3 tomatoes
100 g (4 oz) bean shoots
100 g (4 oz) white cabbage or chinese leaves
salt and pepper

1. Mix together the sesame oil, soy sauce, vinegar and honey with 1 tablespoon water. Peel and crush the garlic and add to the mixture. Cut the tofu into 2.5 cm (1 inch) dice and place in the marinade. Leave for at least 1 hour in the refrigerator.
2. In the meantime, trim, wash and chop the celery. Trim, clean and slice the mushrooms. Peel and coarsely chop the tomatoes. Rinse the bean shoots and drain well. Finely shred the white cabbage or chinese leaves.
3. Transfer the prepared salad ingredients to a salad bowl. Just before serving, add the tofu and the marinade to the salad and mix carefully together. Season with salt and pepper to taste.

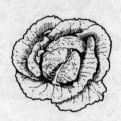

MEXICAN TOFU AND BEAN STEW

Serves 4
Cooking time 25–30 minutes

1 x 275 g (10 oz) packet tofu
1 large onion
2–3 cloves garlic or 1½ teaspoons garlic paste
1 small green pepper
1 small red pepper
1–2 tablespoons oil
2 teaspoons ground cumin
1 teaspoon ground coriander
1–2 teaspoons chilli powder or to taste
1 tablespoon lemon juice
1 teaspoon sugar
1 x 400 g (14 oz) can chopped tomatoes
1 tablespoon tomato purée
1 x 400 g (14 oz) can red kidney beans
225 g (8 oz) cooked or canned chick peas
300 ml (10 fl oz) vegetable stock
salt
2 teaspoons arrowroot
chopped fresh coriander or parsley, to garnish

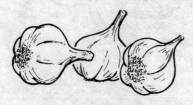

1. Cut the tofu into large dice and leave to drain on kitchen paper.
2. Peel the onion and garlic. Chop the onion and crush the garlic. Remove the stalks, pith and seeds from the peppers and cut into small dice.
3. Heat 1 tablespoon oil in a heavy pan and cook the tofu until

lightly coloured. Remove from the pan. Add more oil if necessary and add the garlic. Cook for a few seconds then add the cumin and coriander. Mix well and cook for about 15 seconds, then add the onion and peppers. Cook gently for about 5 minutes, stirring occasionally so that the spices do not stick to the pan.

4. Stir in the chilli powder, lemon juice and sugar with the chopped tomatoes and tomato purée. Drain and rinse the beans and chick peas and add to the pan with the stock and the tofu. Bring to the boil and season to taste. Lower the heat and cook for 15–20 minutes until the onions and peppers are tender.

5. Mix the arrowroot with a little water and add to the pan. Bring to the boil, stirring all the time. Check the seasoning and pour into a hot serving dish. Just before serving, sprinkle the chopped coriander or parsley over. Serve hot.

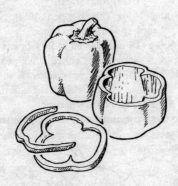

SMOKED TOFU KEBABS

Serves 4
Cooking time 7–10 minutes plus marinading overnight

2 x 275 g (10 oz) packets naturally smoked tofu
2 tablespoons olive oil
3 tablespoons Worcestershire Sauce
3 tablespoons soy sauce
2 tablespoons lemon juice
1/2 teaspoon black pepper
1 large green pepper
1 large red pepper
16 small mushrooms
16 small tomatoes or 8 larger ones
salt

1. Cut each block of tofu into 16 pieces. Heat the oil in a pan or wok and cook the tofu until it is golden brown on all sides. Remove from the pan and place in a shallow dish.
2. Mix together the Worcestershire Sauce, soy sauce, lemon juice and black pepper. Pour over the tofu. Cover and leave to marinate in the refrigerator overnight.
3. On the following day, remove the tofu pieces from the marinade. Remove the stalks, pith and seeds from the peppers and cut into long strips. Clean and trim the mushrooms and cut larger tomatoes (if used) in half. Blanch the peppers in boiling, salted water for 3–4 minutes. Drain well and cool under cold running water.
4. Fold the pepper strips into three and thread on to skewers, alternating with the tofu, mushrooms and tomatoes, and allowing two kebabs per person. Cook on a barbecue or under a hot preheated grill until the vegetables are cooked. Brush frequently with the marinade whilst they are cooking.
5. Serve hot on a bed of rice with a side salad if desired.

Salads and Vegetables

Readers of the first *Hip and Thigh Diet Cookbook* will know how popular the Oven Chips (page 195) became so I make no apologies for including them for readers who have not seen the recipe before. I have also included a variation on Oven Sauté Potatoes (page 196) and another old favourite, Dry Roast Potatoes (page 194).

This chapter contains lots more ideas for tasty and attractive salads and a good selection of other vegetables to add colour and flavour to your meals. Some of the salads can also be used as starters or lunch dishes, and the Potato Quiche (page 191) can be also used as a lunch or supper dish as well as an accompaniment to other dishes.

Mange-tout may seem expensive but only small amounts are needed which makes them less of the luxury they may at first seem. Simple vegetables such as cauliflower and cabbage are given a new flavours and for something different, try the Hot Vegetable Salad (page 197). I love celeriac, both cooked and grated raw in a salad. If you have never tasted it, do try the Celeriac Paysanne (page 198). Do try it also in a purée with potatoes (page 204) which is delicious with roasts and stews.

Readers who are looking for a dainty and decorative accompaniment should try the Courgette and Carrot Timbales (page 202). They are surprisingly easy to make and look so attractive and impressive. Whether you want a recipe for family meals or for entertaining, I am sure you will find plenty to satisfy you.

Salads and Vegetables

> (V) suitable for vegetarians
> (B) budget-conscious recipe
> (Q) quick to prepare and cook

BEAN AND MUSHROOM SALAD

Serves 4–6

225 g (8 oz) fresh bean sprouts
2 carrots
100 g (4 oz) button mushrooms
6 spring onions
25 g (1 oz) raisins, optional
6 tablespoons low-fat fromage frais or low-fat natural yogurt
¼ teaspoon chilli powder
1–2 teaspoons soy sauce
1 teaspoon clear honey
1 tablespoon lemon juice
salt and white pepper

1. Wash and drain the bean sprouts. Peel and grate the carrots.
Trim, wash and slice the mushrooms and spring onions. Mix
together in a salad bowl with the raisins, if used.
2. Whisk together the fromage frais or yogurt, chilli powder,
soy sauce, honey and lemon juice. Season to taste with salt and
pepper, adding a little more chilli powder or soy sauce to taste.
Mix well, pour over the salad and refrigerate until required.

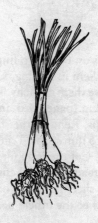

GOURMET SALAD WITH KIWI SAUCE

Serves 4–6

4 medium courgettes
4–5 tomatoes
1 small green pepper
1 small red pepper
1 head fennel (approximately 200 g (7 oz)) or celery sticks
6 spring onions
4–5 kiwi fruit
2 tablespoons sherry
1 tablespoon lemon juice
2 teaspoons honey
1 egg yolk
4 tablespoons low-fat natural yogurt
salt and white pepper
1 lettuce

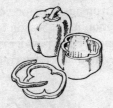

1. Trim the courgettes and cut into finger-length batons. If you wish you can blanch them in boiling, salted water for 2–3 minutes but I prefer to leave them crunchy. Drain them well and chill under the cold tap. Skin (page 246) and de-seed the tomatoes. Cut the flesh into strips. Remove the stalk, pith and seeds from the peppers and cut into thin strips. Trim the feathery leaves from the fennel and reserve. Cut the bulb into quarters and slice thinly. If celery is used instead, trim and cut into finger-length strips and reserve. Trim and slice the spring onions. Peel the kiwi fruit. Chop 2 coarsely and slice the others neatly.

2. Press the chopped kiwi fruits through a nylon sieve. If you wish you can first purée them lightly in a food processor. Place the sherry, lemon juice and honey in a small bowl with the egg yolk. Place over a pan of hot water and beat until thick. Remove from the heat and stir in the yogurt and the puréed kiwi fruits. Season to taste with salt and white pepper.

3. Wash and drain the lettuce. Roll the leaves up a few at a time, like a cigar and cut into thin strips. Mix together the lettuce, peppers, fennel or celery and the spring onions. Pile on to a serving dish. Arrange the courgette fingers and the strips of tomato on the top with the kiwi fruit around the edge. Cover and refrigerate until required.

4. Just before serving, whisk the sauce well and pour over the salad. Sprinkle some chopped reserved fennel leaves over the top.

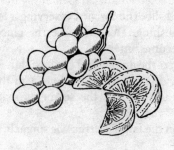

CHICORY AND APPLE SALAD

Serves 4

Lamb's lettuce or small spinach leaves both have a slightly sharp taste which contrasts very well with the other ingredients. If you cannot get either of them use the leaves of small cos (Little Gem) or some other decorative lettuce.

2 heads chicory
1 red apple
1 green apple
1 orange
100–175 g (4–6 oz) lamb's lettuce or small spinach leaves
3–4 tablespoons Low-fat Salad Cream (page 238) or
Oil-free Vinaigrette (page 239)

1. Trim, wash and slice the chicory, reserving a few of the smaller leaves for garnishing. Do not leave the chicory soaking in water or it will become bitter.
2. Core and quarter the apples and cut into thin slices. The skins are left on to provide a contrast in colour. Cut the peel and pith from the orange and cut out the segments from between the membranes.
3. Wash and drain the lamb's lettuce or spinach. Place in a salad bowl.
4. Mix together the chicory, apples and orange with the Low-fat Salad Cream or Oil-free Vinaigrette. Refrigerate until required and pile on top of the lettuce just before serving.

ORANGE AND ONION SALAD

Serves 4

Red-skinned onions are best for this recipe as they look so attractive and are mild in taste. If you cannot buy these use any other mild onions, such as Spanish.

350 g (12 oz) red-skinned onions
3 medium oranges
2 tablespoons white or red wine vinegar
4 tablespoons sherry
2 teaspoons clear honey
salt and black pepper
chopped dill or parsley, to garnish

1. Peel and thinly slice the onions. Cut the peel and pith from the oranges and slice them thinly.
2. Whisk together the wine vinegar, sherry and honey. Season to taste with salt and black pepper.
3. Mix the oranges and onions together in a bowl. Pour on the dressing and mix well. Cover and refrigerate until required. Sprinkle the dill or parsley over before serving.

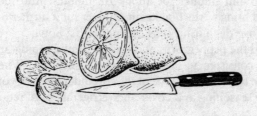

MUSHROOMS À LA GREÇQUE

Serves 4

Although this dish is usually cooked with olive oil and white wine in the Greek fashion, you will find this recipe just as tasty. It is an excellent accompaniment to cold meats or you could serve in individual ramekins as a starter.

2 lemons
1 tomato
6–8 small pickling onions
350 g (12 oz) small button mushrooms
200 ml (7½ fl oz) white wine or cider
1 teaspoon coriander seeds
6–8 black peppercorns
2 teaspoons tomato purée
1 bay leaf
salt and black pepper

1. Squeeze the juice from one lemon. Cut the other in half and then quarter each piece. Skin the tomato (page 246) and quarter. Peel the onions. Trim and clean the mushrooms.
2. Put all the ingredients except the mushrooms into a pan, bring to the boil and simmer for about 10 minutes. Add the mushrooms and bring to the boil again, simmer for a further 6–7 minutes. Remove the mushrooms and put into a bowl.
3. Discard the peppercorns and boil the liquid rapidly until it is a coating consistency. Pour over the mushrooms. When cold, remove the bay leaf and some of the coriander seeds (if you wish). Check the seasoning and cover and refrigerate until required.

FARMER'S-STYLE MANGE-TOUT

Serves 4
Cooking time 20–25 minutes

175 g (6 oz) carrots
1 medium onion
100 g (4 oz) mange-tout
4–5 lettuce leaves
2–3 sprigs parsley
2–3 sprigs chervil
300 ml (10 fl oz) chicken or vegetable stock
salt and black pepper
1/2 teaspoon arrowroot
chopped parsley and/or chervil, to garnish

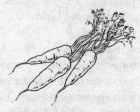

1. Peel and finely slice the carrots and onion. Top and tail the mange-tout. Remove any coarse stalks from the lettuce leaves. Roll the lettuce leaves up like a cigar and cut into thin shreds.
2. Place the onion in a pan with the parsley and chervil sprigs and the stock and simmer for about 10 minutes. Add the carrots and cook for another 2–3 minutes then add the mange-tout and the lettuce. Cook for another 5 minutes or until the mange-tout are tender but still have a 'bite'. Remove the vegetables, taste and season with salt and pepper if necessary. Cover and keep hot. Discard the parsley and chervil sprigs. Boil the stock to reduce it to 150 ml (5 fl oz). Mix the arrowroot with a little water and add to the pan. Bring to the boil, stirring all the time. Pour over the vegetables and sprinkle the chopped herbs over the top just before serving. Serve hot.

SPICED CAULIFLOWER

Serves 4
Cooking time 12–15 minutes

1 small onion
15 g (1/2 oz) fresh root ginger
1 teaspoon coriander seeds
2 teaspoons mustard seeds
1 lemon
1 cauliflower
1/2 teaspoon chilli powder
1/2 teaspoon turmeric
chopped fresh coriander or parsley, to garnish

1. Peel and grate the onion and 1–2 teaspoons of ginger. Crush the coriander and mustard seeds. Grate the lemon rind and squeeze the juice from the lemon.
2. Break the cauliflower into small florets and cook in boiling, salted water for 8–10 minutes or until just tender.
3. Place the onion, ginger, coriander and mustard seeds in a small pan together with the grated rind and juice of the lemon, the chilli powder and turmeric. Add 3 tablespoons water and cook for 3–4 minutes
4. Drain the cauliflower well and return to the pan. Pour the spice mixture over and toss lightly. Place in a hot serving dish and sprinkle coriander or parsley over just before serving. Serve hot.

POTATO QUICHE

Serves 4
Cooking time 40–45 minutes
Oven 200°C, 400°F, Gas Mark 6

This vegetable quiche is an ideal accompaniment to grilled and cold meats and can also be served as a lunch dish with salad. The ham can be omitted if it is served as a vegetable or vegetarian dish.

450 g (1 lb) old potatoes
1–2 tablespoons skimmed milk
2 tablespoons flour
salt and black pepper
350 g (12 oz) carrots
2 tablespoons low-fat fromage frais or low-fat natural yogurt
1 egg
pinch nutmeg
175 g (6 oz) mushrooms
3 tomatoes
100 g (4 oz) lean ham, optional
2–3 tablespoons fresh breadcrumbs
2–3 teaspoons Parmesan cheese (maintenance dieters
and vegetarians only)

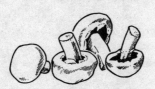

1. Peel the potatoes and cut into evenly sized pieces. Cook in boiling, salted water for 15–20 minutes until tender. Drain well. Mash until smooth with the milk and the flour and season to taste with salt and pepper. Place in the bottom of a 18 cm (7 in) non-stick loose-bottomed flan tin or a lightly oiled quiche dish. Press out with a spoon to form a flan shape.

---

2. Meanwhile, peel and slice the carrots and cook in boiling, salted water until tender. Drain well then purée in a food processor or liquidizer with the fromage frais or yogurt and the egg. Season to taste with salt and pepper and a pinch of nutmeg. Pour into the potato case.

3. Wash, trim and slice the mushrooms. Skin (page 246) and slice the tomatoes and chop the ham (if used). Sprinkle the ham over the carrots, cover with the sliced mushrooms and then with the tomatoes. Season lightly and sprinkle the breadcrumbs over the top. Maintenance dieters and vegetarians can mix a little Parmesan cheese with the breadcrumbs. Place in a preheated oven at 200°C, 400°F, Gas Mark 6 for 25–30 minutes until the potato is golden and the mushrooms are cooked. Serve hot.

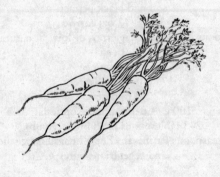

ITALIAN VEGETABLE CASSEROLE

Serves 4
Cooking time 20–25 minutes

1 large onion
1 large green pepper
1 large red pepper
3 courgettes
4 tomatoes
100 g (4 oz) mushrooms
2–3 cloves garlic or 1–1½ teaspoons garlic paste
300 ml (10 fl oz) chicken or vegetable stock
1 tablespoon tomato purée
salt and black pepper
1 teaspoon arrowroot
1–2 tablespoons low-fat fromage frais or low-fat natural yogurt
chopped parsley or basil, to garnish

1. Peel and chop the onion. Remove the stalk, pith and seeds from the peppers and cut the flesh into large dice. Trim the courgettes and cut into thick slices. Skin (page 246), de-seed and chop the tomatoes. Trim and clean the mushrooms and cut in halves or quarters according to size. Peel and crush the garlic.
2. Place the onion in a pan with the stock and simmer until almost tender, then add the peppers, courgettes, tomatoes, mushrooms, garlic and the tomato purée. Season to taste and cook for a further 5–7 minutes until all the vegetables are tender.
3. Remove the vegetables and keep hot. Mix the arrowroot with a little water and add to the pan. Bring to the boil, stirring all the time. If the sauce is too thick add a little more stock or water and reheat. Add the fromage frais or yogurt and reheat gently but do not boil. Replace the vegetables and check the seasoning. Pour into a hot serving dish and sprinkle parsley or basil over the top just before serving. Serve hot.

DRY ROAST POTATOES

Serves 3–4
Cooking time 1–1¼ hours
Oven 200°C, 400°F, Gas Mark 6

450–550 g (1–1¼ lb) medium old potatoes
salt

1. Peel the potatoes and cut into evenly sized pieces if you wish.
Place in a pan of cold water, bring to the boil and blanch for 5
minutes.
2. Drain thoroughly then lightly scratch the surface of each
potato and sprinkle lightly with salt.
3. Place on a non-stick baking tray without any fat and bake in
a preheated oven at 200°C, 400°F, Gas Mark 6 for about 1–1¼
hours.

OVEN CHIPS

Serves 4
Cooking time 35–45 minutes
Oven 220°C, 425°F, Gas Mark 7

2–3 large old potatoes
1 teaspoon oil

1. Peel the potatoes and cut into chips. Blanch in boiling, salted water for 5 minutes. Drain well.
2. Meanwhile, pour the oil on to a baking sheet and place in a preheated oven at 220°C, 425°F, Gas Mark 7 for 7–10 minutes until the oil is very hot.
3. Spread the chips over the baking tray and turn them gently until they are coated with oil.
4. Bake for 35–45 minutes (depending on the size of the chips) until they are soft in the middle and crisp on the outside. Turn them once or twice during the cooking time.

OVEN SAUTÉ POTATOES

Serves 3–4
Cooking time 45–50 minutes
Oven 220°C, 425°F, Gas Mark 7

This is a variation of Oven Chips which were so popular in the last *Hip and Thigh Diet Cookbook*.

450–550 g (1–1¼ lb) small old or new potatoes
1 teaspoon oil

1. Peel or scrape the potatoes and cook in boiling, salted water for 10 minutes. Drain well and slice thickly.
2. Heat the oil and cook in the same way as Oven Chips (page 195).

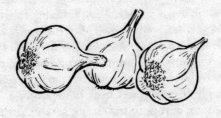

HOT VEGETABLE SALAD

Serves 4
Cooking time 10–12 minutes

225–350 g (8–12 oz) small new or firm old potatoes
4 medium carrots
2 medium courgettes
225 g (8 oz) broccoli
1 clove garlic or ½ teaspoon garlic paste
2 medium tomatoes
8 tablespoons Oil-free Vinaigrette (page 239)
salt and black pepper
chopped herbs of your choice, to garnish

1. Wash the new potatoes and if you wish scrape them. Peel the old potatoes and the carrots. Trim the courgettes. Slice or dice the potatoes and cut the carrots and courgettes into thick slices. Trim and wash the broccoli and break into small florets.
2. Peel and crush the garlic. Skin (page 246) and de-seed the tomatoes and cut them into moderately small dice.
3. Mix the garlic with the vinaigrette.
4. Cook the potatoes and carrots in boiling, salted water for 5–8 minutes until nearly tender. Add the courgettes and broccoli and cook for a further 3–4 minutes until the broccoli and courgettes are just tender. Drain well, cover and keep hot.
5. Just before serving, pour the vinaigrette into the pan and heat through without boiling. Stir in the tomatoes quickly and return the vegetables to the pan. Check the seasoning. Toss well in the hot vinaigrette and pour into a hot serving dish. Sprinkle some herbs over and serve immediately.

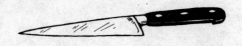

CELERIAC PAYSANNE

Serves 4–6
Cooking time 40–50 minutes

Celeriac is a root vegetable which resembles a rough creamy-brown swede but tastes like celery. When buying celeriac press the roots hard to make sure they are firm because they can be soft and spongy inside. Peel them thickly like swede and, if you are not cooking them immediately, keep them in water with a little lemon juice or vinegar until they are required. This will prevent them discolouring. Left-over stock and vegetables can be puréed to form the basis of a very tasty soup. If you are unable to obtain celeriac, use extra celery.

1 small celeriac, approximately 350–450 g (12 oz–1 lb)
4–6 small onions
4–6 small carrots
3–4 sticks celery
450 ml (15 fl oz) chicken or vegetable stock
salt and black pepper
chopped parsley, to garnish

1. Peel the celeriac and cut into 2–2.5 cm (3/4–1 inch) cubes. Peel the onions and carrots and cut into quarters or slice the carrots thickly. Wash and trim the celery and cut into short lengths.
2. Place the vegetables in a pan with the stock. Bring to the boil and simmer very gently for 40–50 minutes until the vegetables are tender.
3. Check the seasoning and pour into a hot serving dish with the cooking liquor. Sprinkle parsley over just before serving. Serve hot.

ORIENTAL CABBAGE

Serves 4
Cooking time 8–10 minutes

This is good served with roast or cold meats.

450–550 g (1–1¼ lb) trimmed cabbage
4 tablespoons red wine vinegar
2 tablespoons brown sugar
1 teaspoon caraway seeds

1. Remove any coarse stalks from the cabbage and shred it very finely. Cook in boiling water for 3–4 minutes. Drain well.
2. Return to the pan with the vinegar and brown sugar. Cover and cook for a further 4–5 minutes until the cabbage is only just tender, then raise the heat to reduce the vinegar. Stir in the caraway seeds, pile into a hot serving dish and serve immediately.

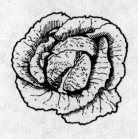

HERBY MASHED POTATOES

Serves 4
Cooking time 20 minutes

This potato dish is excellent with salads. Omit the eggs and the ham if it is served with a main course. Vegetarians may also like to use this recipe, omitting the ham.

450–550 g (1–1½ lb) old potatoes
2–3 tablespoons skimmed milk or low-fat natural yogurt
salt and black pepper
1–2 hard-boiled eggs
100 g (4 oz) lean ham, optional
1 medium onion
1 tablespoon chopped chives
1 tablespoon chopped parsley
½ teaspoon dried oregano

1. Peel the potatoes, cut into evenly sized pieces and cook in boiling, salted water until tender. Drain well. Mash and cream well with the milk or yogurt. Season to taste with salt and black pepper.
2 Peel and chop the hard-boiled eggs and cut the ham into small dice, if used. Peel and grate the onion. When the potatoes are ready, stir the onion in with half the chopped chives and parsley, all the oregano and the ham, if used.
3. Pile into a hot serving dish and sprinkle the chopped egg and the remainder of the herbs over just before serving. Serve hot.

PROVENÇALE MARROW

Serves 4
Cooking time 25–30 minutes

1 medium marrow
2 medium onions
2 cloves garlic or 1 teaspoon garlic paste
1 x 400 g (14 oz) can chopped tomatoes
salt and black pepper
2 teaspoons chopped fresh or dried basil

1. Peel the marrow, cut into half lengthways and remove the seeds. Cut into 2.5 cm (1 in) cubes. Peel the onions and garlic. Finely chop the onion and crush the garlic.
2. Place the marrow in a pan with the onions, garlic and the tomatoes. Season to taste with salt and pepper. Stir in 1 teaspoon of basil and simmer gently until all the vegetables are tender. Check the seasoning. Pour into a hot serving dish and sprinkle a little more basil over the top (if you wish) just before serving. Serve hot.

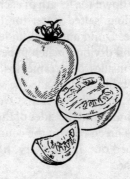

COURGETTE AND CARROT TIMBALES

Serves 4
Cooking time 40–50 minutes
Oven 180°C, 375°F, Gas Mark 5

These timbales look very attractive when used as a garnish, either on a serving dish or, particularly, on individual plates. They can be cooked at the same time as a roast or other dish or can be pre-cooked and reheated in the oven in a roasting tin of hot water at 180°C, 375°F, Gas Mark 5 for 15 minutes.

2 medium carrots, total weight approximately 165 g (5½ oz)
1 medium courgette, approximately 165 g (5½ oz)
50 g (2 oz) quark or other low-fat soft cheese
1 egg
salt and white pepper

1. Trim the carrots and courgettes. Peel the carrots. Using a mandolin or potato peeler, cut 8 thin slices of courgette and 8–10 thin slices of carrot down the length of each vegetable. Blanch the carrot slices in boiling, salted water for 1–2 minutes until they are soft and pliable. Drain and chill under cold running water. Drain well again and dry on kitchen paper.
2. Lightly oil the insides of 4 ramekins. Allowing any excess length of each vegetable to overhang the sides, place one slice of carrot in the centre of each ramekin. Overlap it with a slice of courgette and continue until the sides of the ramekin are covered. Make certain that a green edge of the courgettes will show when the ramekin is turned out. If necessary, fill in any gaps with the extra slices of carrot.
3. Slice the remaining carrot and courgette. Cook the carrot for 5–6 minutes in boiling, salted water, until tender. Drain well. Chill as above. Blanch the courgette for 1 minute only. Chill, drain and dry on kitchen paper.

---

4. Purée the carrot and the courgette separately in a food processor or vegetable mill, adding 25 g (1 oz) quark or other low-fat soft cheese to each mixture. Whisk the egg well and stir half into each vegetable. Season each one well to taste.

5. Place a layer of the carrot purée into each prepared ramekin and cover with the other purée. Fold the excess strips over the top and press down lightly.

6. Place in a roasting tin of boiling water and cover lightly with aluminium foil. Cook in a preheated oven at 180°C, 375°F, Gas Mark 5 for 40–50 minutes until they are firm to touch. Turn out of the ramekins and serve hot.

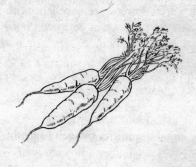

VEGETABLE PURÉES

Vegetable purées have become very popular in recent years. Individual vegetables can be used or you can combine two together. I find them useful because they can be prepared in advance and either reheated in a microwave oven or covered and heated in a conventional oven in a roasting tin of boiling water. All the vegetables are boiled first in the normal way unless otherwise stated. The quantities given assume that other vegetables are served with the purées. If you wish, a little quark or other low-fat soft cheese or low-fat fromage frais or low-fat natural yogurt can be beaten into each purée. Purées are excellent with all roast and grilled meats. Left-over purées can be frozen but I prefer not to freeze the Celeriac and Potato Purée.

CARROT
450 g (1 lb) *serves 4–6*

CARROT AND PARSNIP
Use equal quantities of each vegetable

450 g (1 lb) *serves 4–6*

CARROTS AND LEEK
225 g (8 oz) carrots
450 g (1 lb) trimmed leeks
serves 4

Drain leeks until they are very dry before puréeing. If the mixture is still too wet, mix 1/2–1 teaspoon arrowroot with a little water, stir into the purée in a small pan and bring to the boil stirring all the time.

CELERIAC AND POTATO
Use equal quantities of each vegetable
450 g (1 lb) *serves 3–4*

This is excellent with all casseroles.

PUMPKIN AND CELERIAC

Use two-thirds pumpkin to one-third celeriac. Cook the pumpkin in skimmed milk.

750 g (1½ lb) pumpkin, weighed before peeling
450 g (1 lb) celeriac, weighed before peeling
serves 4–6

SWEDE
450 g (1 lb) *serves 4–6*

JERUSALEM ARTICHOKE
450 g (1 lb) *serves 4–6*

SPLIT PEA

Soak split peas in cold water overnight then drain and place in a pan with a sliced onion, carrot and bay leaf. Cover with water and bring to the boil. Simmer for 1½–2 hours until the peas are tender. Drain, reserving the liquid which can be used for soup and discard the bay leaf. Purée the peas in a food processor or vegetable mill. Season to taste with salt and pepper and add a little of the cooking liquor, if necessary, to give a smooth consistency. For Pease Pudding, use yellow split peas, see page 146. Traditionally served with Boiled Beef (page 145).

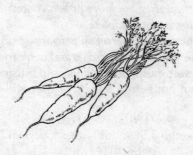

CRISPY COURGETTES

Serves 4–6
Cooking time 25–30 minutes
Oven 200°C, 400°F, Gas Mark 6

450 g (1 lb) courgettes
2–3 tablespoons flour
salt and black pepper
2–3 egg whites
2–3 tablespoons reduced-oil low-calorie salad dressing,
e.g. Waistline or Weight Watchers
5–6 tablespoons fresh breadcrumbs
1 teaspoon oil

1. Trim the courgettes and cut each one in 2–3 finger-length pieces. Cut each piece in half and each half into two or three batons.
2. Put the flour in a plastic bag and season well with salt and black pepper. Whisk the egg whites until they are light and frothy and stir into the salad dressing. Pour into a shallow dish. Place the breadcrumbs in another plastic bag.
3. Place a handful of the courgette batons into the flour. Close the top and shake well. Remove and pass them a few at a time through the egg-white mixture and then shake them in the bag of breadcrumbs until they are more or less coated. It does not matter if the coating is not complete.
4. To cook them, heat the oil in a roasting tin in a preheated oven at 200°C, 400°F, Gas Mark 6 and cook for 25–30 minutes until they are soft on the inside and crisp outside. Do not cover if keeping them hot before serving or they will lose their crispness and soften.

Desserts

Whoever thought a cheesecake could be part of a diet? Just look at the Pineapple and Lemon Cheesecake (page 219). Turn a simple pineapple into another dish fit for a king, see Pineapple Folly (page 210), or learn how to make meringues in a few seconds in your microwave.

All these dishes and many more wait for you to try, from a Strawberry and Passion Fruit Pavlova (page 231) to simple Grape and Mint Jelly (page 216), quick and easy Orange and Honey Bananas (page 222), or colourful Peaches Aurora (page 221). I have also included a recipe for a *cake*, Sultana Bran Cake (page 215). I have said in the recipe that it can be stored for up to a week but you will be lucky if your family lets it last so long unless you hide it.

All the recipes in this section are very low in fat and cautious with calories and can be eaten by all dieters as part of their main meal of the day.

Desserts

Ⓥ suitable for vegetarians
Ⓑ budget-conscious recipe
Ⓠ quick to prepare and cook

APRICOT AND GINGER FOOL

Serves 4

1 x 400 g (14 oz) can apricot halves in natural juice
450 g (1 lb) quark or other low-fat soft cheese
1 tablespoon syrup from a jar of stem ginger
2–3 pieces stem ginger
a few mint leaves, to decorate

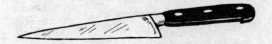

1. Drain the apricots and purée the fruit in a food processor or liquidizer with the quark or other low-fat soft cheese and the ginger syrup. Transfer to a bowl.
2. Chop the stem ginger and fold most of it into the apricot mixture. Taste and add more stem ginger to your own taste. Reserve a little for decoration. Chop this more finely.
3. Spoon the mixture into individual glasses, cover and chill in the refrigerator until required. Wash and dry the mint leaves. Just before serving, place a little of the reserved chopped ginger on the top of each one and decorate with one or two small mint leaves.

PINEAPPLE FOLLY

Serves 4–6

225 g (8 oz) fresh or frozen blackcurrants
2–3 tablespoons sugar or artificial sweetener to taste
$1/2$ teaspoon arrowroot
1 medium pineapple
4 kiwi fruit
100 g (4 oz) seedless grapes
7–8 strawberries
2–3 tablespoons rum or other liqueur, optional
low-fat fromage frais or ice cream, optional

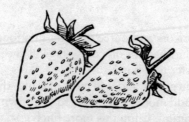

1. Cook the blackcurrants in 8 tablespoons of water until they are tender. Sweeten to taste with sugar or artificial sweetener. Purée the blackcurrants lightly in a food processor or liquidizer. Take care to work the machine for only a moment or two to break up the skins. If you work it for too long, the seeds will make the sauce gritty. Using a nylon sieve to prevent the purée discolouring, press the blackcurrants well against the sides of the sieve with a wooden spoon so that all the purée is extracted from the seeds. Return the purée to a clean pan. Mix the arrowroot with a little water and add to the pan. Bring to the boil, stirring all the time. Taste and add more sugar or sweetener if desired. Pour into a bowl or sauceboat and stir from time to time to prevent a skin forming on the surface. This sauce freezes well.
2. Cut the pineapple in half through the leaves and, using a grapefruit knife, cut the flesh away from the skin. Remove the

centre core with a sharp knife and cut each pineapple half into 6 slices.

3. Peel and slice the kiwi fruit. Wash the grapes and cut the strawberries in half.

4. Place the slices of kiwi in the pineapple shells and arrange the sliced pineapple on top, round side uppermost. Arrange the grapes around the edge and half a strawberry at the top and bottom of each shell and between each slice. Cover well with food wrap and refrigerate until required. If you wish, a little rum or liqueur can be poured over the pineapple.

5. To serve, arrange the pineapple shells on a large plate and serve the sauce separately. Fromage frais or ice cream can also be served with the pineapple.

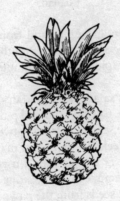

SPICED TROPICAL SALAD

Serves 4–6

4 small oranges
3 tablespoons light brown soft sugar
$1/2$ teaspoon cinnamon
3–4 tablespoons rum or to taste
50 g (2 oz) fresh dates
2 kiwi fruit
1 ripe mango
1 ripe pawpaw or 2 peaches
1 small pineapple
4–5 lychees
1 star fruit, optional
1 banana

1. To make the syrup: grate the rind from 2 oranges. Dissolve the sugar in 6 tablespoons of water with the cinnamon and grated orange rind. Boil rapidly for 3–4 minutes. Cool and then add the rum.

2. To make the fruit salad: skin the dates, cut each one in half and remove the stone. Cut the rind and pith from all the oranges and either remove the segments from between the membranes or cut into thin slices. Peel the kiwi fruit, mango and pawpaw (or pour boiling water over the peaches if used and leave for a few minutes then peel). Remove the large stone from the centre of the mango, scoop out the seeds from the pawpaw or the stones from the peaches, if used.

3. Cut the skin from the pineapple. Cut in half and cut out the hard core, then cut the flesh into dice. Dice the mango and pawpaw and slice the kiwi and peaches, if used.

4. Peel the lychees and cut each one in half. Slice the starfruit, if used. Put all the fruit in a bowl and pour over the syrup. Cover and refrigerate for 2–3 hours.

5. Just before serving, slice and add the banana. Serve chilled.

GRAPEFRUIT AND KIWI DESSERT

Serves 4–6

One of the fascinating things about cookery is that there is always something new to learn or to surprise you. I was certainly surprised when testing this recipe to find that not only was the jelly containing the kiwi fruit not setting, it was reverting to a liquid. I realized that kiwi fruit must contain an enzyme called papain, which is also found in fresh pawpaws and pineapple and will dissolve any animal protein. As papain has this characteristic, it is the basis of most meat tenderizers and because gelatine is a form of animal protein it will be attacked by papain. However, it is easy to overcome as papain is killed by heat so if the fruit is blanched for a minute or two in boiling fruit juice it can then be set in jelly. Vegetarian or vegan readers using gelatine substitutes based on carrageen or agar-agar will not need to blanch the kiwi fruit: it is only gelatine, derived from animals, which is affected.

600 ml (1 pt) ruby red unsweetened grapefruit juice
7 level teaspoons powdered gelatine
75 g (3 oz) sugar or artificial sweetener to taste
3–4 kiwi fruit
2 large pink grapefruit
1 orange
225 g (8 oz) low-fat cottage cheese
300 ml (10 fl oz) low-fat natural yogurt
2 egg whites

1. Take 3 tablespoons of grapefruit juice and place in a small bowl. Sprinkle 3 teaspoons gelatine on to the juice and leave to soften, then stand it over a pan of hot water until it dissolves completely. Measure out 450 ml (15 fl oz) of grapefruit juice and mix with the dissolved gelatine. Sweeten to taste with sugar or artificial sweetener. Pour a little into the base of an 18 cm (7 in) non-stick tin or soufflé dish or a 20 cm (8 in) ring mould. Stand

---

the tin or dish in a pan of cold water and ice (page 245) and leave to set.

2. Peel the kiwi fruit and cut into 25 mm ($^1/_8$ in) slices. Reserve 4 tablespoons of the remaining grapefruit juice and put the rest into a small pan with the sliced kiwi fruit. Bring to the boil and cook for a few moments, then drain and allow to cool. Discard the juice (you could save it for use in a fruit salad).

3. Grate the rind from one of the grapefruits and the orange, taking care not to grate any of the pith as this will be bitter. Cut the peel and pith from both grapefruits and the orange and cut out the segments from between the membranes. Reserve any juice. Cut each segment into 2 or 3 pieces.

4. Arrange some kiwi slices decoratively on top of the set jelly. Pour on a little more jelly and leave to set. Cover with the remainder of the kiwi slices and pour on the remainder of the jelly. Refrigerate until set.

5. Place the reserved 4 tablespoons of grapefruit juice in a small bowl. Sprinkle the remainder of the gelatine on top and dissolve as before.

6. Purée the cottage cheese and yogurt with the grated grapefruit and orange rinds until smooth then pour into a large bowl. Stir in the dissolved gelatine and the chopped fruit. Season to taste with sugar or artificial sweetener. Stand in water and ice, as before, until it is on the point of setting.

7. When the mixture is firm enough to hold a trail from a spoon, whisk the egg whites until they stand in stiff peaks. Fold them into the mixture carefully with a metal spoon or spatula.

8. Pour on to the jelly and refrigerate until set. To serve, turn out on to a round plate.

SULTANA BRAN CAKE

Makes 8–10 1 cm (¹/₂ in) slices
Cooking time 45–55 minutes
Oven 180°C, 350°F, Gas Mark 4

This is a very easy cake to make and is ideal for use on the Hip and Thigh Diet because it contains no fat. Do remember that it must be left to soak overnight before baking. This cake keeps well in an airtight tin or sealed plastic box for several days. It also freezes well.

75 g (3 oz) All Bran or similar shredded bran
225 g (8 oz) sultanas
100 g (4 oz) dark brown soft sugar
300 ml (10 fl oz) skimmed milk
200 g (7 oz) self-raising flour

1. Line a 450 g (1 lb) tin with greaseproof paper or use a non-stick tin.
2. Place the All Bran, sultanas and sugar into a bowl and pour on the milk. Cover and refrigerate overnight.
3. The next day, add the self-raising flour and mix well together. Spoon into the prepared tin. Bake in a preheated oven at 180°C, 350°F, Gas Mark 4 for 45–55 minutes, until a skewer inserted in the cake comes out clean.
4. Leave until cold, then remove the paper. When quite cold, place in a plastic bag or airtight tin to store.
5. Maintenance Dieters can spread a little low-fat spread, jam or honey on a slice of cake if they wish but will probably find that it is just as delicious without.

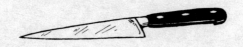

GRAPE AND MINT JELLY

Serves 4

1 packet lime jelly
300 ml (10 fl oz) apple juice
2 tablespoons crème de menthe
225 g (8 oz) seedless green grapes
1 tablespoon clear honey or to taste
150 ml (5 fl oz) low-fat fromage frais or low-fat natural yogurt
a few small mint leaves, to decorate

1. Dissolve the jelly in 250 ml (8 fl oz) water. Stir in the apple juice and leave until cool then add the crème de menthe.
2. Remove the stalks from the grapes and, if you wish, remove the skins by pouring boiling water over them. Leave for a few minutes, drain and cover with cold water, then peel.
3. Reserve a few grapes for decoration and divide the remainder between 4 glasses. When the jelly is on the point of setting pour it over the grapes. Leave it until set.
4. Warm the honey until it is runny and stir into the fromage frais or yogurt. Pour over the jelly and decorate the top of each jelly with the reserved grapes and 1 or 2 mint leaves. Chill until required.

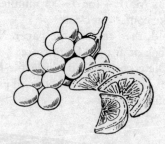

APPLE AND MANDARIN DELIGHT

Serves 4

450 g (1 lb) cooking apples
1 1/2 teaspoons lemon juice
1/4 teaspoon ground ginger
225 ml (7 1/2 fl oz) low-fat fromage frais or low-fat natural yogurt
1 tablespoon sugar or artificial sweetener to taste
3 teaspoons powdered gelatine
1 x 225 g (8 oz) can mandarin segments in natural juice
2 egg whites

1. Peel, core and slice the cooking apples and cook in a pan with 3–4 tablespoons water until soft. If the apples are still juicy, cook them a little longer, stirring them all the time until the surplus juice evaporates. Purée the apples in a food processor or liquidizer with the lemon juice and ground ginger. Stir in the fromage frais or yogurt and sweeten to taste with sugar or sweetener.
2. Pour 3 tablespoons water into a small bowl, sprinkle on the gelatine and leave to soften. Place the bowl over a pan of boiling water and stir until the gelatine is dissolved. Add to the apple mixture.
3. Drain the mandarin oranges. Reserve a few segments for decoration and stir the remainder into the apple mixture.
4. When the mixture is on the point of setting, whisk the egg whites until they stand in stiff peaks and fold in carefully using a metal spoon or spatula. Pour into individual glasses or a larger dish and decorate with the reserved mandarin slices when it is set. Serve chilled.

FRUIT SNOWBALLS

Serves 4
Cooking time 35–45 minutes
Oven 200°C, 400°F, Gas Mark 6

4 medium cooking or Golden Delicious apples
(or Williams or Comice pears)
1 tablespoon lemon juice
a little sugar or artificial sweetener, optional
1 tablespoon currants
1 tablespoon chopped peel
1–2 tablespoons ginger marmalade, optional
2 egg whites
100 g (4 oz) castor sugar

1. Peel and core the apples or pears and place the fruit in a deep casserole dish. Pour on 300 ml (10 fl oz) water and brush the fruit with lemon juice. Sprinkle a little sugar or sweetener over each one if you wish. Cover and cook in a preheated oven at 200°C, 400°F, Gas Mark 6 for about 30 minutes or until the fruit is tender. Take care not to overcook the apples. Pears will take a little longer.

2. When the fruit is cooked, lift it from the casserole, drain well then place on an ovenproof serving dish. Fill the centres of the apples with the currants and chopped peel. Pears can be stuffed with this mixture or with ginger marmalade.

3. To serve, raise the oven temperature to 230°C, 450°F, Gas Mark 8. Whisk the egg whites until they stand in stiff peaks. Fold the sugar in carefully in three batches. Coat each apple or pear with the meringue and return to the oven for 5–8 minutes or until the meringue is golden brown. Serve immediately.

PINEAPPLE AND
LEMON CHEESECAKE

Serves 4–6
Cooking time 30–40 minutes
Oven 160°C, 325°F, Gas Mark 3

A cheesecake in a diet book was a challenge I couldn't resist. The topping was easily adapted from the first cheesecake recipe I ever made but inventing a fatless base for a cheesecake proved rather difficult. After several experiments I had the idea for the one I have given in this recipe and I hope you will like it. This is best if you assemble it just before serving so that the base remains crisp. If you pre-prepare the decoration it takes only a moment or two to transfer to the top of the cheesecake. Although using both egg whites in the cheesecake makes it much lighter, if you want to economise you can use one egg white in the cheesecake and use the other one for the base.

1 x 400 g (14 oz) can pineapple slices in natural juice
1 x 11 g (1/2 oz) packet gelatine
1 lemon
225 g (8 oz) low-fat cottage cheese
150 ml (5 fl oz) low-fat natural yogurt
2 eggs
50 g (2 oz) castor sugar
50 g (2 oz) icing sugar
1 extra egg white
40 g (1 1/2 oz) porridge oats
a few strawberries, to decorate

1. Line the base of an 18 cm (7 in) loose-bottomed cake tin or deep sponge tin with greaseproof or silicone paper.
2. Drain the pineapple slices and reserve 4 tablespoons of the juice. Save two pineapple rings for decoration and chop the remainder coarsely.

3. Sprinkle the gelatine on to the reserved pineapple juice and leave to soften, then stand the bowl over a pan of hot water and stir until the gelatine has dissolved completely.

4. Grate the rind and squeeze the juice from the lemon.

5. Place the cottage cheese and yogurt in a food processor or liquidizer with the grated lemon rind. Work until smooth then pour into a large bowl. Add the chopped pineapple to the food processor or liquidizer and process until the pineapple is finely chopped. Stir into the cottage cheese and yogurt mixture.

6. Separate the eggs. Whisk the egg yolks with the castor sugar and lemon juice in a bowl over a pan of hot water until they thicken. Mix together with the cottage cheese and pineapple mixture and the gelatine. Place the bowl in another bowl filled with ice and water (page 245) and let the mixture almost set.

7. When the mixture is on the point of setting, whisk the egg whites until they stand in stiff peaks and fold into the mixture. Pour into the prepared tin and leave in the refrigerator until set.

8. To make the base, first of all draw a circle (slightly smaller than the base of the tin you are using) on the underside of a sheet of silicone paper and place it on a baking sheet. Mix the icing sugar and the extra egg white together in a bowl and place it over a pan of gently steaming water. Whisk until the mixture stands in stiff peaks. Remove from the heat and gently fold in the porridge oats. Spread over the marked circle on the silicone paper and cook in a preheated oven at 160°C, 325°F, Gas Mark 3 for 30–40 minutes until the base is crisp. Remove from the oven and cool, then peel off the paper.

9. Just before serving place the meringue base, rough side down, on top of the cheesecake. Turn out on to a round serving plate and decorate around the top with the reserved pineapple slices which have been cut into pieces and the strawberries.

FREEZING

The cheesecake can be frozen and the base made and stored separately in an airtight container. Defrost in a refrigerator.

PEACHES AURORA

Serves 4–6
Cooking time 15–20 minutes

50 g (2 oz) granulated sugar
6–8 ripe peaches
450 g (1 lb) strawberries or raspberries
1 tablespoon lemon juice
1 teaspoon arrowroot
low-fat fromage frais or low-fat natural yogurt, to serve
castor sugar or sweetener to taste

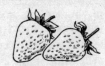

1. Place the sugar with 300 ml (10 fl oz) water in a frying-pan. Cover and simmer until the sugar has dissolved.
2. Halve the peaches, remove the stones and place skin side up in the syrup. Poach gently for 15–20 minutes, turning the peach halves over half-way through the cooking time. Lift the peaches from the pan and remove the skins. Place on a wire rack to drain and cool.
3. In the meantime, reserve a few strawberries or raspberries for decoration and purée the remainder of the fruit lightly in a food processor or liquidizer, then sieve through a nylon sieve to remove the pips. Place the purée in a pan with the lemon juice and bring to the boil. Mix the arrowroot with a little water and add to the pan. Return to the boil, stirring all the time. Sweeten to taste with castor sugar or sweetener. Cool, stirring occasionally to prevent a skin from forming.
4. When the peaches and purée are cold, pour the purée into a shallow serving dish. Carefully arrange the peaches on top and decorate the dish with the reserved strawberries. Cover and refrigerate until required. Serve chilled with fromage frais or yogurt.

ORANGE AND HONEY BANANAS

Serves 4
Cooking time 15–20 minutes
Oven 200°C, 400°F, Gas Mark 6

2–3 oranges
4 firm bananas
2 tablespoons honey
1/4 teaspoon cinnamon
2 tablespoons Grand Marnier or rum, optional
low-fat fromage frais or low-fat natural yogurt, to serve

1. Grate the rind and squeeze the juice from 2 of the oranges. If you wish to decorate the dish when it is completed, decorate the other orange with a canelle knife (page 245) if you like, and cut it into thin slices. Cut each slice in half and reserve.
2. Peel the bananas and cut them in half lengthways. Place them in an oven-to-table dish.
3. Place the rind and juice of the oranges in a pan with the honey and cinnamon. Heat through until the honey has dissolved. Pour over the bananas and cover the dish with aluminium foil. Cook in a preheated oven at 200°C, 400°F, Gas Mark 6 for 15–20 minutes.
4. Remove from the oven and stir in the Grand Marnier or rum (if used). Serve hot with fromage frais or yogurt.

AUSTRIAN APPLE AND ORANGE RING

Serves 6

3 oranges
1 lemon
425 ml (15 fl oz) orange juice
75 g (3 oz) granulated sugar
1½ x 11g (½ oz) sachets of gelatine
4 Golden Delicious or similar eating apples
2–3 tablespoons rum, optional
low-fat fromage frais or low-fat natural yogurt, to serve

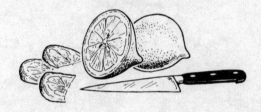

1. Peel the rind very thinly from 2 oranges, using a potato peeler. Cut into very fine (julienne) strips. Grate the rind of the lemon. Squeeze the juice from these oranges and the lemon and make up to 600 ml (1 pint) with the extra orange juice. Add a little water if necessary to give the required amount. Cut the rind and pith from the remaining orange and cut out the segments from between the membranes or, if you prefer, cut the orange into thin slices and cut each slice in half. Reserve the segments or slices for decoration.

2. Place the strips of orange rind and grated lemon juice in a pan with 150 ml (5 fl oz) water and simmer gently until tender. Add the sugar and stir until it has dissolved.

3. Place 4 tablespoons of the orange and lemon juice in a small bowl. Sprinkle the gelatine on the surface and leave for a few

minutes to soften. Then place the bowl over a pan of hot water and stir until the gelatine has dissolved. Stir the gelatine and syrup into the juice with the orange and lemon rind.

4. Peel, core and grate the apples and stir into the orange jelly. Taste and if necessary add a little more sugar or artificial sweetener to taste. Pour into a 20 cm (8 in) ring mould and refrigerate until set.

5. To serve, dip the ring mould into hot water for 3–4 seconds then unmould on to a round serving plate. Decorate with the reserved orange. Serve with fromage frais or yogurt.

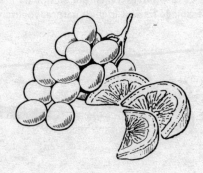

MICROWAVE MERINGUES

Cooking time 1 minute 40 seconds. (This time applies to a
600-watt microwave. Adjust the timing if your microwave has
a higher or lower wattage.)
Makes 32

It is only possible to make meringue discs with this recipe but
they are ideal for serving with sorbets, ice cream or fruit.

1 egg white
275 g (10 oz) icing sugar

1. Lightly whisk the egg white until it is frothy.
2. Sift the icing sugar on to the egg white a little at a time to form
a stiff paste. You will find it easier to use your hand in the later
stages. Divide the paste into four and cut each quarter into eight.
Form each piece into a round ball.
3. Cut a circle of silicone paper the same size as the turntable in
your microwave. Place one ball in the centre of the paper and the
others evenly around the edge. Cook on high for 1 minute 40 seconds. Take the paper and meringues from the oven, cool for a
moment or two then remove the meringues. Repeat until all the
mixture is used. Store in an airtight container until required.

FRUIT TERRINE

Serves 6

I first ate this terrine in the south-west of France near Agen, an area renowned for its apricots and plums. The apricots were very ripe and juicy but you may find the apricots you buy are a little too firm to purée easily. In this case, poach 225 g (8 oz) of apricots in a little sugar syrup or extra orange or apple juice. This juice can then be used in the apricot jelly.

350 g (12 oz) strawberries
350 g (12 oz) apricots (fresh or canned)
350 g (12 oz) raspberries
75–100 g (3–4 oz) icing sugar or artificial sweetener if desired
1½ x 11 g (½ oz) packets gelatine
12 tablespoons white wine or orange or apple juice
4–5 kiwi fruits
1 lemon

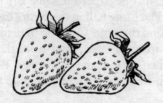

1. Hull and purée 225 g (8 oz) strawberries. Slice the remainder of the strawberries. Do the same with the apricots and raspberries, keeping each group separate. Sieve the strawberries and raspberries through a nylon sieve to remove the pips and seeds. Sweeten each purée with 1 tablespoon of sugar or artificial sweetener to taste.

2. Pour 2 tablespoons of water into each of three small bowls. Divide the gelatine into 3 and sprinkle one portion into each bowl. Leave until soft, then place one bowl over hot water and stir until it has dissolved. Mix it into the strawberry purée with 3 tablespoons of white wine, orange or apple juice. Add the sliced

strawberries and pour into a 750 g–1 kg (1¹/₂–2 lb) tin or mould. Stand this in a bowl containing ice and water (page 245) and leave until set.

3. Repeat with the apricot purée, adding it to the bowl of strawberry purée. When that is set do the same with the raspberry purée. Refrigerate until required.

4. Peel, purée and sieve the kiwi fruit. Squeeze the juice from the lemon and stir into the purée. Place in a pan and boil for 2–3 minutes. Add sugar or sweetener to taste. Cover and refrigerate until required.

5. To serve, dip the mould into hot water for 4–5 seconds and turn out on to a serving dish. Serve the kiwi fruit sauce separately.

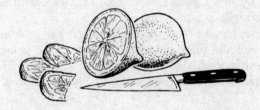

PEACH YOGURT ICE

Serves 4

1 x 400 g (14 oz) can peach slices in natural juice
l00 g (4 oz) castor sugar
600 ml (1 pint) low-fat natural yogurt
l quantity Raspberry Sauce (page 244)
extra canned peach slices, optional

1. Drain the juice from the can of peaches into a small pan. Add the sugar and heat gently until the sugar has dissolved. Allow to cool.

2. Purée the peach slices in a food processor or liquidizer and add the juice and the yogurt. Place in a l litre (2 pint) plastic box (or two 500 ml (1 pint) boxes). Seal each box with a lid and freeze overnight or until required.

3. To serve, remove from the freezer about half an hour before it is required and place in the refrigerator. Place scoops of the yogurt ice in individual dishes, pour a little Raspberry Sauce over and decorate with some chopped peach slices if desired.

LEMON AND RASPBERRY MERINGUES

Serves 4

If you wish you can use a bought lemon sorbet but you will find the one on page 230 very simple to make.

4 meringue nests or 8 Microwave Meringue discs (page 225)
Lemon Sorbet (page 230)
1 quantity Raspberry Sauce (page 244)

1. Fill the meringue nests with lemon sorbet or sandwich two discs together with a good scoop of sorbet. This can be done in advance and returned to the deep freeze until required. Take from the deep freeze and place in the refrigerator for 10–15 minutes before serving.
2. Place the meringues on a serving dish or individual dishes and pour a little Raspberry Sauce over each one. Serve the rest of the sauce separately.

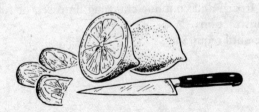

LEMON SORBET

Serves 6–8

4 large juicy lemons
225 g (8 oz) granulated sugar
1 egg white

1. Wash the lemons and pare the rinds very thinly using a potato peeler. Make certain that no pith remains on the peel or the
sorbet will be bitter. Squeeze the lemons and make the juice up
to 750 ml (1¼ pints) with water.
2. Place the rinds, liquid and sugar in a pan and heat gently until
the sugar has dissolved. Cover, chill and leave for 6–8 hours or
overnight.
3. Strain the rind from the liquid and discard. Place the liquid in
a sealed plastic box in the freezer or in an ice-cream maker.
4. If using a plastic box then, when the mixture is lightly frozen,
remove it from the freezer and beat well with an electric hand
whisk until it is smooth. Repeat this two or three times, adding
the lightly whisked egg white on the last occasion. If you are
using an ice-cream maker, add the egg white when the mixture
is lightly frozen and continue churning until set, or follow the
maker's instructions.
5. Freeze until required.

STRAWBERRY AND PASSION FRUIT PAVLOVA

Serves 8
Cooking time 1½–2 hours
Oven 110°C, 225°F, Gas Mark ¼

Use size 3 eggs for this recipe to give you the right amount of egg white. Ripe passion fruit feel heavy and have a dark wrinkled skin. They are filled with seeds (which are edible) and juice and have a delicious aroma. If possible, remove the seeds and pulp from the passion fruit just before you serve this pavlova so that this lovely aroma is appreciated by your guests.

250 g (9 oz) castor sugar
1 tablespoon cornflour
4 egg whites
2 teaspoons white wine vinegar
½ teaspoon vanilla essence
225–450 g (8 oz–1 lb) low-fat fromage frais
4–6 ripe passion fruit
225–350 g (8–12 oz) small strawberries

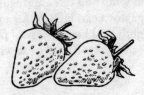

1. Draw a 20 cm (8 inch) circle on the underside of a sheet of silicone paper. Place on a baking sheet.
2. Sieve the castor sugar and cornflour together.
3. Whisk the egg whites at high speed in a large bowl until they stand in very stiff peaks. Whisk in one-third of the sugar and cornflour for about a minute until the egg whites are stiff again and no grains of sugar can be seen. Whisk half the remaining

sugar into the egg whites in a similar manner and repeat with the rest of the sugar. Continue whisking until the egg whites are very thick and smooth.

4. Sprinkle the white wine vinegar and vanilla essence over the meringue and whisk in very quickly.

5. Pile the mixture on to the prepared silicone paper. Using a palette knife, spread the meringue out over the marked circle and form it into a flat cake shape about 7.5 cm (3 inch) thick. Bake in the centre of a preheated oven at 110°C, 225°F, Gas Mark 1/4 for 1 1/2– 2 hours. If you are using a fan-assisted oven, use the lowest setting. It may be necessary to reduce the cooking time.

6. When the pavlova is golden brown and firm to the touch, remove it from the oven and place on a wire rack to cool. When it is completely cold, loosen it away from the paper with a palette knife. Place a plate lightly on the top. Turn over and carefully peel off the paper.

7. About 1–2 hours before the pavlova is required, spread the fromage frais over the surface. Just before serving cut the passion fruit in half and scoop out all the seeds and pulp. Spread them over the centre of the pavlova and decorate around the edge with whole or halved strawberries. If you want to prepare the passion fruit in advance, place the seeds and pulp in a small bowl, cover very tightly with food wrap and refrigerate until required.

8. The base of this pavlova can be kept for up to 2 days before it is used. Cover it lightly and keep in a cool place. Do not place in a tin or refrigerator to store it because it will go soft.

Sauces and Salad Dressings

One of the most difficult things to do when creating a new diet cookbook is to provide a selection of different flavours. In the recipes I have tried to vary these as much as possible but, so often, a sauce is needed as an accompaniment. Tomato sauces are always popular so I have included the Tomato Sauce (page 235) given in the first *Hip and Thigh Diet Cookbook* but I have also given another using fresh tomatoes, Fresh Tomato Sauce (page 236). I have also included some sauces, Spicy Raisin Sauce (page 241), Cumberland Sauce (page 242) and Fromage Frais and Horseradish Sauce (page 240), which will enhance your grilled, boiled and roast meats.

Salads so often need a dressing to make them more appealing so, apart from the original Oil-free Vinaigrette (page 239), try the tangy Tomato Oil-free Dressing (page 237). If you still yearn for a salad cream, try my recipe for Low-fat Salad Cream. It is adapted from a recipe I have had for many years which used soured cream. The yogurt makes a very acceptable substitute.

Sauces

(V) suitable for vegetarians

(B) budget-conscious recipe

(Q) quick to prepare and cook

TOMATO SAUCE

Makes about 300 ml (10 fl oz)
Cooking time 25–30 minutes

This sauce is quickly made and freezes well so it is useful to make several quantities at one time and freeze them. If you prefer a smooth sauce, use 300 ml (10 fl oz) tomato passata instead of canned tomatoes. Then, when the sauce is cooked, purée it in a food processor or liquidizer or through a vegetable mill. Add stock or water, following the recipe (step 4).

1 medium onion
1–2 cloves garlic or 1/2–1 teaspoon garlic paste
1 x 400 g (14 oz) can chopped tomatoes
salt and freshly ground black pepper
good pinch granulated sugar
1 teaspoon lemon juice
vegetable stock or water as necessary

1. Peel the onion and fresh garlic. Finely chop the onion and crush the garlic.
2. Place the onion and garlic in a pan with the tomatoes (including the juice from the can). Season lightly with salt and freshly ground black pepper and add the sugar and lemon juice.
3. Bring to the boil and simmer gently, uncovered, for 25–30 minutes until the onion is tender.
4. Check the seasoning, adding more salt, pepper, sugar or lemon juice as required. Dilute the sauce with stock or water, if necessary, to give a pouring consistency.

FRESH TOMATO SAUCE

Makes about 300 ml (10 fl oz)
Cooking time 20–25 minutes

This sauce freezes well and is ideal to make if you have a glut of tomatoes in the garden.

550 g (1¼ lb) ripe tomatoes
1–2 cloves garlic or ½–1 teaspoons garlic paste
150 ml (5 fl oz) chicken or vegetable stock
salt and black pepper
good pinch sugar
1 teaspoon lemon juice
vegetable stock as necessary

1. Cut the tomatoes into quarters. Peel and crush the garlic.
2. Place the tomatoes in a small pan with the stock and garlic. Season lightly with salt and black pepper and add the sugar and lemon juice. Simmer gently for about 20 minutes.
3. Press the tomatoes through a wire sieve with a wooden spoon, pressing the skins well against the sides of the sieve to extract all the sauce possible. Dilute with more stock, if necessary, to give a coating consistency, then check the seasoning and add more salt, pepper, sugar or lemon juice to taste.

TOMATO OIL-FREE DRESSING

Makes 225 ml (7 1/2 fl oz)

1 pickling onion or 1 clove of garlic or 1/2 teaspoon garlic paste
1 tablespoon chopped basil or parsley, optional
150 ml (5 fl oz) tomato juice
4 tablespoons red wine vinegar
2 teaspoons Worcestershire Sauce
1 tablespoon soy sauce
1 teaspoon French mustard
salt and black pepper

1. Peel the onion or garlic. Finely chop the onion or crush the garlic.
2. Combine all the ingredients except for salt and pepper in a screw-top jar or a plastic container with a lid. Shake vigorously until well mixed. Taste and season with salt and pepper if required.
3. Store in the refrigerator and use as required.

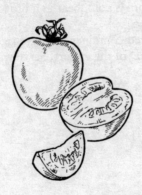

LOW-FAT SALAD CREAM

Makes approximately 225 ml (7 1/2 fl oz)

2 teaspoons castor sugar
2 teaspoons flour
1 teaspoon dry mustard
1 teaspoon salt
pinch cayenne pepper
5 tablespoons malt vinegar
1 egg yolk
150 ml (5 fl oz) low-fat natural yogurt
skimmed milk to dilute

1. Mix the sugar, flour, mustard, salt and cayenne pepper in a small pan, preferably not aluminium, and stir in the vinegar. Mix until smooth, then beat in the egg yolk. Bring to the boil over a gentle heat, stirring all the time and cook for 1–2 minutes, still stirring.
2. Remove from heat and stir in the yogurt. Leave until cold, beating occasionally to prevent a skin from forming.
3. When the mixture is cold, beat in a little milk to give a thick pouring consistency.
4. Store in a covered container in the refrigerator for 4–5 days or until 'use-by date' of the yogurt. Serve with salads, coleslaw, etc.

OIL-FREE VINAIGRETTE

Makes 200 ml (7 fl oz)

You can make up this amount of dressing in advance and store
it in the refrigerator ready for use when required. Use either the
chopped fresh herbs or the garlic to give additional flavour.

150 ml (5 fl oz) white wine vinegar or cider vinegar
50 ml (2 fl oz) lemon juice
1/2 teaspoon salt
1/2 teaspoon freshly ground black pepper
3–4 teaspoons castor sugar
11/2 teaspoons French mustard
chopped fresh herbs such as thyme, marjoram,
basil or parsley, optional
1 crushed clove garlic or 1/2 teaspoon garlic paste, optional

1. Mix all the ingredients together, pour into a screw-top jar or
other container with a tight-fitting lid and shake well. Taste and
add more salt, black pepper or sugar if you wish.
2. Store in the refrigerator and shake well before using.

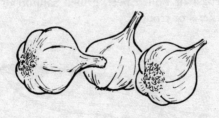

FROMAGE FRAIS AND HORSERADISH SAUCE

Makes approximately 250 ml (8 fl oz)

It is possible to buy grated horseradish in jars or you can grow it in the garden and peel and grate it yourself. Do take care not to get the juice of the horseradish anywhere near your eyes as it is very pungent. Wash your hands carefully after using it. If grated horseradish is not available, use a proprietary brand of horseradish relish. A hot one is best.

200 g (7 oz) low-fat fromage frais
2 tablespoons grated horseradish or horseradish relish
1 tablespoon lemon juice
salt and white pepper

1. Mix the fromage frais with 1 tablespoon grated horseradish and the lemon juice. Season with salt and white pepper. Taste and add more horseradish to suit your taste.
2. Cover and leave in a refrigerator for 2–3 hours to allow the flavour to develop.
3. This sauce will keep for 4–5 days, covered in a refrigerator. Serve with roast or boiled beef, grilled salmon or chicken, or smoked mackerel or trout.

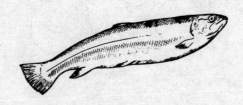

SPICY RAISIN SAUCE

Makes approximately 350 ml (12 fl oz)

This sauce freezes well so you may wish to make up several
batches at the same time.

75 g (3 oz) stoned raisins
2 cloves
1/2–1 teaspoon ground cinnamon
75 g (3 oz) brown sugar
1–1 1/2 teaspoons arrowroot
salt and black pepper
1 tablespoon lemon juice

1. Place the raisins, cloves and the cinnamon in a saucepan with
300 ml (10 fl oz) water. Bring to the boil and simmer for 10 minutes.

2. Add the sugar and stir until it has dissolved. Mix the arrowroot with a little water and add to the pan. Season with salt and
pepper and add the lemon juice. Bring to the boil, stirring all the
time.

3. Remove from the heat, remove the cloves and leave the sauce
for about 30 minutes to allow the flavours to develop.

4. Reheat and serve with liver, lamb, gammon steaks or boiled
bacon.

CUMBERLAND SAUCE

Makes approximately 225 ml (7¹/₂ fl oz)

1 orange
1 lemon
4 tablespoons redcurrant jelly
4 tablespoons port
2 level teaspoons cornflour

1. Peel the rind thinly from the orange and lemon, using a potato peeler. Cut the rind into very thin (julienne) strips. Place in a
pan, cover with water and simmer for 5 minutes.
2. Squeeze the juice from the orange and lemon. Place in another pan with the redcurrant jelly. Simmer gently until the jelly has
dissolved, stirring occasionally.
3. Add the port to the juices and jelly mixture. Mix the cornflour
with a little water and add to the pan. Bring to the boil, stirring
all the time and boil for 2–3 minutes (still stirring) until the sauce
thickens and clears.
4. Drain the orange and lemon rind and stir into the sauce.
5. This sauce will keep in a covered container in the refrigerator
for 4–5 days. Serve with ham or pork.

THREE-VEGETABLE FONDUE

This sauce was made to accompany the Vegetable Terrine (page 153) but will make an excellent dressing for all salads.

Makes approximately 225–300 ml (7¹/₂–10 fl oz)

225 g (8 oz) ripe tomatoes
50 g (2 oz) red pepper (weighed without pith or seeds)
25 g (1 oz) onion or shallot
2 small cloves garlic or 1 teaspoon garlic paste
1 tablespoon red wine vinegar
3 tablespoons vegetable or chicken stock
salt and pepper

1. Skin (page 246) and de-seed the tomatoes. Place the flesh in a sieve and press out as much juice as possible. Cut the pepper into pieces. Peel and coarsely chop the onion or shallot and garlic.
2. Purée the vegetables with any tomato juice, the vinegar and stock in a liquidizer or food processor until they are smooth.
3. Strain the sauce and season to taste with salt and pepper. Cover and refrigerate until required. Use within 2–3 days.

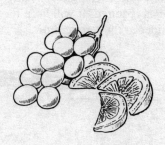

RASPBERRY SAUCE

Makes approximately 275 ml (7½ fl oz)

This sauce freezes very well so when raspberries are plentiful and at their cheapest you can, if you wish, make a quantity of this sauce and freeze it in small quantities.

175–225 g (6–8 oz) fresh or frozen raspberries
2–3 teaspoons icing sugar or to taste
1–2 teaspoons lemon juice, optional
1 scant teaspoon arrowroot

1. Place the raspberries in a small pan with 3–4 tablespoons water. Simmer for 3–4 minutes then add icing sugar and lemon juice to taste.
2. Sieve the raspberries through a nylon sieve (a metal one will discolour the raspberries) and stir and press the seeds well against the sides of the sieve with a wooden spoon to extract all the pulp possible.
3. Make sure there are no seeds in the pan and return the sauce to it. Bring to the boil. Mix the arrowroot with a little water and add to the pan. Bring to the boil, stirring all the time. Pour into a bowl and leave to cool, stirring occasionally to prevent a skin from forming. Use as required. It will keep for 6–7 days if kept in a covered container in the refrigerator.

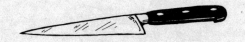

USEFUL HINTS AND TIPS

CANELLE KNIFE

This is a special knife with a V-shaped blade and is used to cut strips from cucumbers, oranges and lemons to give a decorative edge.

CHILLING GELATINE MIXTURES

Whenever the recipe instruction is given to chill gelatine mixtures to enable them to set, you will notice I always say to place in a bowl or pan of ice and water. This will chill the mixture far more rapidly than putting its bowl directly on ice as the cold conducted by the water completely surrounds the dish or mould. If ice alone is used, only the parts in contact with the ice are chilled.

DRY-FRYING AND FRYING-PANS

Any heavy-based frying-pan will be suitable for dry-frying. It will be helpful to have one with a lid as some recipes call for this. To brown the meat for any stews, make certain that the pan is really hot before you begin cooking. Test with one piece of meat. It should seal the outside immediately. If the pan is not hot enough, the juice will seep out and the result will be tough, colourless meat. Cook it in several batches. Too much turning or stirring will allow the meat to cool and the juices to run out of the meat. Add liquid to the pan and, with a wooden spatula, mix in any juices which have caramelized in the pan so that this extra colour and flavour is not wasted.

Vegetables can also be browned without fat. Make certain that the pan is hot, add the vegetables then lower the heat slightly so that the vegetables brown slowly but do not scorch. Stir them occasionally so that they colour evenly. If you wish to soften the vegetables, cover them with a lid and lower the heat when they are lightly browned. It takes a little time to brown vegetables in this way but it will be well worth the time spent as it does add extra flavour to your stews and casseroles.

FROMAGE FRAIS

Fromage frais is used frequently in this book. It consists of skimmed milk and lactic acids and is made with two different fat contents. The low-fat variety has only 0.1 per cent and one grocery chain states that 'it is virtually fat-free'. The other fromage frais has cream added to it and has a fat content of 8 per cent. Only the low-fat fromage frais should be used in the recipes in this book.

Take care when using fromage frais in sauces. Heat it gently; it must not boil as it will curdle if overheated. For this reason, sauces are best made on the cooker, not in a microwave.

REFRESHING

One instruction frequently given in the recipes is to chill cooked or blanched vegetables under cold water until completely cold. This is called refreshing and the reason for chilling the vegetables in this way is to preserve the colour and flavour. It keeps green vegetables bright and prevents vegetables such as potatoes and cauliflower from turning black. It also prevents the strong flavour of a cold cooked vegetable developing. This is particularly important when cooking cauliflower and Brussels sprouts for re-use.

SKINNING TOMATOES

Make sure that the tomatoes are ripe. Using the point of a small, sharp knife, remove the stalk end of the cores. Plunge the tomatoes into boiling water for 30 seconds, then immediately transfer them to cold water and leave to stand until completely cold. This will prevent the flesh of the tomatoes becoming mushy. The skins will then slip off easily.

Index